PARTNERS IN
HEALING

What to Say, Do and Give
When a Friend is Sick

Belsie González, MPH

With
Roberto González Rivera

This book is intended as a reference volume only, and is not intended to take the place of medical or psychological treatment or counseling. If you suspect you need psychological help, seek the services of a mental health professional. The American Psychological Association can help. Visit https://locator.apa.org.

Cover design by Roberto Gonzalez Studio.
Author photo by KapturaElMomento.com.

Dedication

To my mother, Helen Rivera, who has given birth to me three times. She brought me to this world when doing so put her life at risk and then brought me back to life twice by the hand of God with dedication and sacrifice. She is my super heroine.

"I slept and dreamt that life was joy. I awoke and saw that life was service. I acted and behold, service was joy."

— Tagore

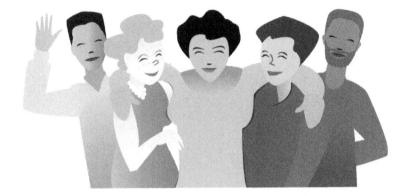

CONTENTS

"It is divinity that shapes, not only your ends, but also your acts, your words and thoughts."

— Swami Sivananda

A Note on Language

In this book I have chosen to use feminine pronouns when speaking about friends or loved ones who may be sick or injured. There is some debate as I write this about whether it is proper to use masculine pronouns when referring to an indeterminate subject. For example, it is usual to say, "Respect the patient's wishes and let *him* lead the way." Some people propose the use of the plural pronoun in these cases. For example, "Respect the patient's wishes and let *them* lead the way." I do not find this elegant. The same goes for the clunky *him/her* combination. Others propose a new, genderless pronoun. I am not that avant-guarde, but neither am I inclined to use masculine pronouns in these cases. I am a woman and I am the author of this book and I prefer to use female pronouns.

Go back to the first sentence of the paragraph above. Reading "friends or loved ones who may be sick or injured" can get tiresome after a few times. This book is for people who have a friend or loved one who is sick or injured (see?) but for economy's sake sometimes you will read "friend," sometimes you will read "loved one." After all, aren't you your loved one's friend? As for her condition, you will usually read "sick." Since my own experiences were with leukemia, you will find references to cancer and cancer treatments. This book is not only about cancer, though. These principles are also meant for you if your loved one is facing a different illness. They also apply if your friend is facing the aftermath of a life-threatening injury.

Doctors refer to us as patients, but we don't look at ourselves this way. We look at ourselves as people, the same as before we were sick. Sometimes it makes more sense to write "patient," but please remember that the human being who is fighting for her life is more than a patient. She is someone you love. In the pages that follow we will explore all kinds of ways you can show that love.

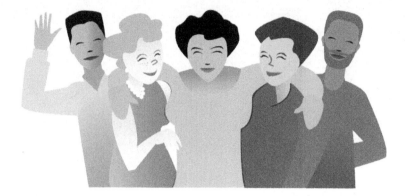

Introduction

I wrote this book for you, the kind friend, coworker or family member whose heart is aching because a loved one is going through a life-threatening disease or recovering from a catastrophic accident. I was once the patient and people like you made my journey to recovery so much better. The following pages describe how.

My goal is to provide you with the practical tools that will help you give the best support you are capable of giving.

"When anxiety was great within me,
your consolation brought me joy."

— Psalm 94:19

My Story, Or How I Became Qualified to Offer This Advice

I am a two-time leukemia survivor.

Without warning my life was turned upside down. I spent my twenty-fifth and twenty-sixth birthdays in different hospitals. I went through chemo with all its attendant horrors. I lost my hair, my dreams, my savings, my identity. I went through a bone marrow transplant. I got well and when I thought I was on my way to accomplishing new dreams, got sick again. At that point a lot of smart and experienced health professionals told me my odds were not good, not good at all. Some were rather discouraging. But the thing is, for all my lovely qualities, there is one thing at which I am not very good. Once I set my eyes on a goal, I'm not good at giving up.

I dried my tears and, with a heart full of faith, I kept fighting.

With the help of the outstanding team at the MD Anderson Cancer Center in Houston, Texas, the mercy of God and my friends and family, I managed to look death in the eye and tell her, *Not now.* That is how I'm here today. I am grateful for every morning. I'm dedicated to helping anyone in any way I can. It's my mission, my duty, my way of thanking God and honoring all the people who helped me

17

when I needed it most. I do it through my work and I do it in my personal life. That is the purpose of this book.

If you are facing a life-threatening illness, I hope you will reach out and create your own support team and make the best use of the resources you have available.

If someone you know is ill or facing the aftermath of a traumatic injury, it can be difficult to know what to say, what to do and what to give. Whether that person is a spouse or a relative, a friend, a co-worker or a neighbor, your words and actions can help or they can hurt. I know, because I have been at the receiving end.

But this book is not only based on my own experiences. It is also based on the experiences of other patients and their friends and relatives who were kind enough to share their stories.

If you're delaying a visit to a sick loved one, don't know what to say to a colleague who has suddenly lost her hair, or if you want to be supportive to your neighbor, the following pages will offer you practical suggestions that will help you turn your good intentions into action. You will learn about:

- Establishing a culture of positivism: the iron rule my brother enforced
- How doing a little something—even once—beats disappearing
- The friend who helped by doing nothing
- Speaking out of love, not fear
- The most common mistake people make (don't be this person!)

Read on to learn what to say, what to do and what to give when someone you love is sick.

*"The best way to find
yourself is to lose yourself
in the service of others."*

— Mahatma Gandhi

Your New Role

You did not sign up for the job, you did not ask for it, but you got it. Someone you know is facing a life-threatening illness or a serious injury. I am sorry you have to go through this. Suddenly you're no longer just the friend or loved one. Now you feel you should have words of wisdom to offer and you have none. You feel people expect you to do something to help and you have no idea what that might be. At the same time, somewhere in the back of your mind, you feel the stab of fear as you realize this person you care about could die. You realize this is out of your control.

You think this must be some kind of misunderstanding. You don't want to think about illness or death. You don't want to lose your friend. You don't want her to suffer, but beneath all that, you are afraid for your own life. The threat to your loved one's life reminds you of your own mortality.

Take a deep breath. It is human nature to think about your own vulnerability when hearing about someone else's. Talk to someone, go for a run, go to the gym. Do whatever works for you, but do not let your fear stop you.

Keep in mind that your friend does not expect you to make the illness disappear. I did not expect that of my friends and family. Neither did any of the survivors who shared their stories with me. Your friend wants you to show up. Your friend wants you to be there, any way you can. You don't need to have all the answers. You don't need to have a collection of deep thoughts about illness and death. Your friend does not expect you to save the day. Be you: the same funny, silly, imperfect, slightly neurotic you they know and love. True, your role will need adjustments. The closer you are to your friend, the more your role will change, but please don't run away.

What you have before you is an opportunity to be kind, to be generous, to be a friend—and you don't have to do it alone.

Help is all around you, and in these pages.

If You Live With Your Loved One

You're bound to feel the effects of your loved one's situation more than most. The illness and treatment will disrupt your home life, your routines and perhaps even your professional life, as you find yourself spending time at hospitals and doctor's offices. You might have to take care of more household chores or find someone who can. This may mean hiring someone or getting help from family members. If children are part of the family, you will want to find the best way to share the news with them. You may have to make new arrangements for child care. If the children are old enough, you may need to get them involved in chores and help them become more self-sufficient. However, remember that they do need emotional support. Reach out to teachers, parents of their best friends, and family members who have bonded with your children. You are not alone in this. When people ask you how they can help, this is one way.

We'll go into more specific ways you can help, but there are a couple of things you will want to do right away.

Inform Yourself

Don't be a passive participant. Do your own research or ask someone you trust to do it for you—maybe a family member or a friend who is good at research or a friend who is a health professional. Take the time to ask questions of your physicians and other healthcare providers. Some doctors are rightly proud of their professional achievements and can come across as arrogant. Don't let that intimidate you. You have a right to understand your treatment options. Ask. If you don't get the answer you need, ask again.

Form Your Team

No one can do this alone. You are in a good position to be the leader of your loved one's support team. This will allow you to coordinate the strategic and tactical support you will need as you face this challenge together. Make sure to build your own support network. You will need it. Your loved one and you will be tested and it is only with guidance and support that you will be your best for your loved one.

Love

Above all, remember your main role is to love. Love through your actions, through silence, through kind words, through patience. Love through taking care of yourself, asking for support. Love through being present even when it is scary.

If You're a Friend or Close Relative

If you're a close friend or relative who doesn't live with the person, you will not find your home life disrupted, at least not to the same extent. This leaves you in a good position to help at your friend's home if you are able. Some ways of doing this may be:

- Preparing occasional meals along with other friends,
- Helping with home repairs,
- Pitching in with household cleaning or sharing the cost of hiring help,
- Picking kids up from school,
- Baby or pet sitting.

Don't wait to for someone to ask you. Offer to do something specific related to your talents or resources.

Even with health insurance, health care expenses will add up. Most people will appreciate any monetary help you can give.

Finally, don't lose sight of your friendship the way it has been up to now. That is what she treasures most of all. Even now that she is fighting for her life, she will need what you have brought to the relationship: your jokes, your fashion skills, your company, just you. You don't need to pretend everything is perfect, but don't focus on the negative, either. More about this later. Your friend is not the illness. Your friend is still your friend.

If You're a Co-Worker

If you're not only a co-worker but also a friend, your role may be like the role described in the previous section. Maybe you only see the patient at work and at work functions. In that case, you may feel awkward about discussing personal health matters. You may feel inclined to say nothing and go about your business. Resist that impulse.

Many people dislike when others over-dramatize the situation. Still, pretending nothing is wrong is not helpful either. Most of us prefer that others acknowledge the illness and at least offer their best wishes. Others will be grateful for prayers. Don't feel the need to offer advice or speak about other people who have been ill. Instead, say something like, "Listen, I'm sorry to hear about your illness. Please accept my best wishes for a speedy recovery."

If your co-worker is in the hospital or home bound, take the time to make a brief call. She may not be able to take the call, but she will appreciate the message. If your co-worker has returned to work, walk up to her, deliver your message and move on. This will actually save you from plenty of awkwardness later. You can even leave a card on her desk with your best wishes. Feel free to include a gift card, if you are moved to do so.

Avoid indulging in office gossip about your co-worker's illness. Patients have enough on their plates. They don't need to deal with office rumors about their health.

On a more practical level, if you can offer specific help with your co-worker's duties, do so. Below you will find some ideas to get you started. Some may not apply to your situation. Be creative.

- Do you have a better parking space? How about switching for a while?
- Speak to your supervisor about taking over part of your co-worker's duties on a temporary basis.
- Donate vacation time, if you have that kind of program at work.
- Offer help with proofreading or editing her reports.
- If you are going out for lunch, offer to bring some back or take her with you.

If You're a Neighbor

Being a neighbor allows you to help in special ways. This depends on the nature of your relationship.

When I was in treatment, my mother had to move to be closer to the hospital. My godmother (and real-life fairy godmother!) took over the care of my mother's house. She handled the mail, paid the bills and looked after the houseplants and the dog and made sure the gardener mowed the lawn and trimmed the bushes. Her help was invaluable to us. You may not be able to do all that, but you may still be able to help. Consider coordinating with other neighbors.

The following list is not meant to be exhaustive. Every situation is different. Reach out to your sick neighbor and to other neighbors and design a plan that works for you.

- If your neighbor lives alone, you may be able to water plants or tend to pets while she is in the hospital or if she doesn't have enough energy to do it herself.

- Mail stacking up in mailboxes or doorsteps may attract the attention of burglars, as it's a sure sign there's no one home. You can offer to pick up your neighbor's mail and keep it for a friend or relative to pick up later.

- You might make sure someone mows your neighbor's lawn. You can do it yourself or you can take over giving instructions to the gardener. You can arrange to have your neighbor send you a check to pay the gardener. If you're in a position to do so, you could take over payments until your neighbor is better. Hospital care is expensive and every little bit counts.

- Keep an eye out for tell-tale signs of leaks or other problems with the house or apartment.

- If your neighbor is away for a long time and they have a car standing idle, it may be good to check the pressure in the car's tires. It can be discouraging to come home to find a car with flat tires. Running it through the car wash may also be a good idea if you have your neighbor's permission.

- If you are authorized to enter your neighbor's home, coordinate with her to have someone come in and clean up.

- Speaking of having access to your neighbor's home, go around and flush the toilets now and then. Rats can hold their breath for a long time. They can swim up pipes and emerge in toilets that have been left unused for a long time. Nobody needs that kind of surprise!

If You're an Acquaintance

If you don't know the patient well and you prefer not to engage personally, that's fine. Sending a card would be a kind gesture, even if it's not extpected. Read the section on What to Say. No one will feel hurt if you say nothing; however, you will probably experience a sense of fulfillment for doing something positive for someone else.

Perhaps you are closer to a friend or relative of the person. In that case, go ahead and offer your good wishes to the person you know. Those who are caring for and supporting the person facing the illness sometimes carry a heavy burden. They deserve acknowledgement and support, too. We will look at this later.

"Love is the capacity to take care, to protect, to nourish."

— Thich Nhat Hanh

WHAT TO SAY

Father Bad News and Other Stories

Shortly after I arrived at the hospital, a priest came around to visit. I was in pain, weak and still trying to wrap my mind around my recent diagnosis. All my hopes and dreams seemed to mean nothing now. Would the cancer kill me, or would the treatment be worse than the disease? My mother, a retired nurse, was all too aware of the dangers of the road before us. She was still in shock and disoriented at finding herself by my bedside in the leukemia ward. The sight of the priest's familiar Roman collar was like a breath of fresh air. Here was someone who would strengthen our faith and give us hope for the future. We welcomed him with smiles.

We were not expecting what happened next.

"A woman in another floor died today," he informed us. "A different kind of cancer. Best thing for her, really, because she had been suffering a great deal at the end. Such a cruel disease!"

Meanwhile, he said, another patient in our floor was not doing well at all. The doctors did not seem optimistic. Her poor mother was heartbroken. Children should not die before their parents. Such a tragedy.

On and on he went, with one tragic tale after another. Every time we interjected a hopeful or positive comment he would nod and barrel on with his pessimism parade. When he finally left we breathed a sigh of relief. Had I had the strength for it, I would have laughed at the sheer lunacy of the scene.

It was not until many years later that I learned that my mother, too, had been ill in her youth. The doctors in my little home town had failed to identify her illness. They could not provide any effective treatment. They had thrown up their hands and commended her to God. A priest had then stared coming in during the afternoons. My mother couldn't stand him.

"I wanted to live," my mother said, "and all he wanted to do was prepare me for death!"

My mother recovered in time. I'm convinced she did it to get back at the priest. I still marvel at the coincidence.

After the priest paid me that first visit, if my mother saw him ambling down the hallway, she would close the door to my room and stand guard outside. If the priest inquired, my mother would claim I was sleeping and excuse herself.

"I'm going to take a little nap while she rests," she would say, closing the door behind her.

"God bless you," the priest would reply. Then he would saunter off to discourage some other unsuspecting soul.

I am happy to say I have also met many Catholic priests who were compassionate and cheerful and full of love. I am grateful for their kindness to this day. The story of Father Bad News is a cautionary tale.

Don't be that guy.

Good intentions count, but they are best when matched with positive actions and words. The things you say can have a great impact on your friend. Use your words to nourish her heart.

Getting the News

If you're reading this book, chances are you already received the bad news that someone you love is sick. You may feel this section is a little late.

But read on.

One of the things people facing a serious illness tell me they do not find helpful is seeing their loved ones break down and cry when they learn of their friend's diagnosis.

When this happens, we tend to feel responsible for the sadness of our loved ones. Your sadness is, of course, understandable. You don't mean to make your friend feel guilty, but this is the human nature we all share. If at all possible, try to moderate your emotional response. If you are close, and she starts crying, you will probably embrace and cry together. That will bring both of you some comfort. Just try to lead the way out of that sadness. Wipe your tears and hers and talk about how you are going to handle this challenge together. Show you care but remember, this moment is about her, not about you.

Be strong. You can allow yourself to break down later.

Is Honesty Still the Best Policy?

You may be wondering if you should be honest with your friend. Should you be all starry-eyed and cheery and pretend everything is wonderful? It depends on what you mean by honest.

The situation is sad, but it won't help us if under the flag of honesty, you are constantly gloomy around us. You may find your friend's physical appearance shocking when you visit. Thinking, "She looks terrible" is natural. Saying "You look terrible" is not nice. Ask yourself, will what I am about to say lift her spirit? Will it make her laugh? How will it show support? If it does not do any of those things, find something else to talk about. Trust me, we are keenly aware of our appearance while going through treatment. It is one of the most difficult things to deal with. We don't have much control of our own body or the way we look, which is a big part of who we are. We are afraid we are losing our lives and the evidence is in the mirror. Whatever you say, make sure it is to help put a positive spin on the situation. You don't need to lie. If your friend asks, remind her that the situation is temporary. You will find a few ideas in the What to Say section.

The same goes for comments about the inevitability of death and the meaninglessness of life. These may be honest, but they are best saved for late-night conversations with other friends at your neighborhood pub.

However, if there is one thing we dislike as much as negative comments it is overly positive ones. We know we are facing a great challenge. Clichés like "This is nothing," or "This will be over in no time" sound hollow, inauthentic, disconnected. We hear such remarks and we feel you are distancing yourself emotionally from us, and no one likes that.

Better to take the middle way. If you can't say something positive and mean it, change the subject. Without prying, ask questions. Talk about other things. Life is still going on. There are many things you can discuss. Honestly.

Dying of Cancer? The Healing Subtleties of Words

My brother met a woman at a café who said her father was dying of cancer.

"Excuse me," he said. "I don't know your father, but it seems to me he is not dying of cancer, but living with cancer. It's a subtle difference, but an important one."

The woman stared at my brother for a moment. Then her face lit up with a smile.

"Oh, my God," she said. "You're right. I had not looked at it that way. It's a small thing, but it does make a difference, doesn't it?"

It does make a difference. It used to be that getting a cancer diagnosis meant the person did not have long to live. That's no longer the case. With new therapies, some people are able to manage their conditions and live for years after their diagnoses. Some of them end up passing away from totally unrelated causes. Others manage to live cancer-free.

While many of the patients I met in my little pink room at the leukemia ward after my first diagnosis passed away, not all did. My friend—let's call her Carmen—is a good example. She was in a room down the hall from me. Today she is healthy and happy and enjoying life. She wasn't dying then and she's not dying now.

Back at the café, my brother continued his conversation. "Neither you nor I know how long your father will be with us," he said. "For all their knowledge and experience, doctors only make educated guesses. They don't know how long a person with cancer will live. Your father may end up living with cancer for many years."

"Actually," the woman said, "he *has* been living with cancer for years now."

"There you go. Was he dying all those years?"

"No. He was living. He's still living."

"Living with cancer."

Belsie González

The Iron Rule

One of my older brothers was living abroad when I received my diagnosis. He immediately quit his job, moved back to look after my mother and me and assumed the responsibility of helping coordinate everything having to do with my treatment. The day after he arrived, unbeknown to me, he stationed himself outside my hospital room, took visitors aside as they arrived and explained the new rule: no more horror stories.

Your friend died of a brain tumor? So sorry. Keep it to yourself.

Your supervisor's wife has breast cancer? So sorry. We don't want to hear about it.

Your aunt died of leukemia? So sorry. Don't talk about it.

He pointed out we were living in the leukemia ward. There were many other patients there. Those patients who were able would visit my room and we would chat. Some of those new friends would not live long. We could not hide from that fact. Furthermore, we knew that life was still going on outside the hospital, with all its wonder and tragedy. We were not blind to life, but he felt I had enough on my plate already. The last thing I needed was more stories of people—

sometimes young people like me—dying of the very illness I was fighting.

My brother was also of the opinion that some people derive an unhealthy pleasure in delivering bad news.

I don't know about that, but I can say one thing: my wonderful friends understood. They were loving and fun.

The horror did not stop. As the days turned into weeks, some the other patients I had met in the ward did, in fact, die. But there were no more stories.

Your friend is not being naive. She knows people get sick and die. She just doesn't want to hear about it right now.

Mind Your Metaphors

A metaphor is a figure of speech in which we apply a word or phrase symbolically. For example, one could say, "I tripped down the staircase of memory." More broadly, it's using something to mean something else.

In her famous essay, *Illness as Metaphor*, Susan Sontag analyzes how harmful certain popular metaphors and myths about illness can be for patients. Don't worry. I am not going to attempt an impersonation of a giant such as Susan Sontag here. Those of you dear readers with a literary inclination can look for Sontag's book. I will, however, say that I believe this: illness does not *mean* anything.

- An illness is not a form of divine judgement.
- Illness is not a punishment.
- Illness is not a reflection of a person's character.
- Being in the company of a person suffering from an illness is not a reflection of your character.
- Being in the company of a person suffering from a non-contagious illness does not contaminate you in any way.

Please save your friend from additional burdens. Do not look at her illness as some kind of metaphor. Refrain from saying anything that may imply that her illness is a punishment for doing something wrong. Even if you strongly believe it is, think about it, how does it help her to learn this now? It is done. According to your belief she is paying the consequences. What are you going to do to ease the journey? Your goal is to help, support, comfort and encourage.

Keep Your Illnesses Straight

In his moving book, *When Your Wife Has Breast Cancer*, Mark S. Weiss tells the story of meeting an acquaintance on the street. The man tells Weiss someone the man knows has died of the same illness that Weiss's wife is battling. When Weiss asks for details, the acquaintance says this other person died of ALS. When Weiss points out that ALS is not cancer, the acquaintance replies that they should find a cure.

Mr. Weiss's acquaintance is right, of course. They should find a cure. In the meantime, while they develop a cure, whoever *they* are, take care not to make the same gaffe.

The man's error suggests a desire to provide support by saying anything that might sound knowledgeable and supportive, when in reality it would have been better to say, "I heard your wife is seriously ill. I am sorry." If you find yourself in a similar situation, offer your well wishes and your help. Don't focus on the diagnosis.

Look inside yourself. If you find fear in your own heart, sit with your fear for a while. Don't try to cover it up or reject it. Feel your fear. Let it wash over you like a wave. Breathe it in and breathe it out and in time you will find some relief. In my present role as one who provides support and not one struggling to stay alive, it helps me to pray and ask for God to guide my words and actions. I also pray for the health of the person who is ill and that immediately brings me peace. Look at your own fears and you will be better prepared to discuss the bad news from a place of compassion. It's more likely that your words will be helpful. You may even feel better about yourself.

There is No One to Blame

We all want to be happy. No one wants to suffer. This seems obvious, but some of the comments we hear when we are sick carry some form of rebuke. Now is not the time to comment on your friend's past nutritional or other habits. Don't mention her weight. Don't talk about where she chooses to live. Don't say anything that she may take as meaning that she has brought her troubles on herself.

Rest assured that your friend's medical team will go over everything she can do to take part in her healing. They will tell her what she should do to improve her chances for a healthy life. Your job is to support your friend now, and scolding doesn't help.

If you believe that we do bring suffering upon ourselves, choose your words with care. If you think that we sign up for certain trials before we are born, please be mindful of the patient's own beliefs. For someone who shares your views, the idea that she chose the illness may bring some comfort. The thought may give her a sense of control. For someone who does not share your views, hearing "This is what you chose" offers no comfort at all. You may find this is a way to wear out your welcome.

Examine your motivations. It may be that finding a cause for the illness, especially one that is not related to your own habits, brings you a false sense of safety. In other words, you may be thinking that the illness happened to your friend because she doesn't have healthy nutritional habits, for example. You then tell yourself that since you have good nutritional habits, it won't happen to you. This helps you feel safe. This is one of those things that makes us human. We like to reassure ourselves. Again, take your time, breathe, hug, ask about how she feels. Let love guide you, not fear.

Live Your Values

This principle arises from the last point in the previous section. If your friend or loved one shares your religious faith and she reaches out to you to strengthen that faith, by all means reach back. However, don't try to help her by persuading her of your religious views. Don't force matters if she has not expressed a desire to discuss the subject with you.

You may feel a sense of urgency to share your view of salvation when someone you love is facing a life-threatening illness, but be wise and gentle. Look out and listen for signs of discomfort. Challenging your friend's values when she is in pain and anguish can be counterproductive. Suggesting that the illness is a sign that she must convert to your religion might bring more fear than comfort and could motivate resistance from some.

Instead, model your beliefs by being respectful and kind to your friend. Embodying your beliefs is the best invitation you can offer another to start a dialog with you. That is, if she wishes to start one. Remember the words of Mahatma Gandhi: *Be the change you wish to see in the world.*

If your friend is not religious and you are unsure of her views, go ahead and ask. If you do, be ready to retreat if she doesn't want to go down that road.

49

You can always pray for her in private or with others.

Do You *Really* Know How They Feel?

No.

You don't.

No, that time you had food poisoning from that burrito doesn't count.

Nor does the time you had that "really bad" cold.

That day you spent vomiting after an all-night bender? Nope.

The same goes for that sob story about when you had chicken pox as an adult.

The only way you may know how a cancer patient or someone with a life-threatening illness feels is if you have faced the same challenge yourself. If that is the case, then your experience is valuable indeed! Many cancer patients report they have found comfort in the stories of survivors. I certainly welcomed the encouragement of cancer survivors when I was fighting for my life.

Since I left the hospital I have had the privilege of sharing my story with other cancer patients. I have found the light of hope in their eyes gratifying. No, not all of them made it, but for a while I gave them a little more hope, a little more strength to fight. Fair warning: not everyone feels the same. I have heard some cancer survivors say they find others who tried to share their experiences irritating. I'm not sure why. In my experience, however, most people welcome that encouragement.

If you are a cancer survivor yourself, I hope you will share the gift of your experience from a positive standpoint. Share how you conquered the fears or the side effects. What helped? What didn't? Just the fact that you are a survivor, that there is life after treatment—hey, even during treatment—will help.

Telling a patient that you know how she feels to establish some kind of bond when you can't back that up is ill-advised.

So unless you have been in the patient's shoes, stay away from this particular cliché. And keep in mind that even if you have had cancer, there are always personal variables that make the experience unique to those going through it. No one really knows how someone else feels. If you are a survivor, listen carefully for similarities with your experiences and share tips to ease the journey and help bring about positive outcomes. I still remember how surprised I was to see someone standing in front of my hospital bed who had gone through the same treatment. It was like looking at a hologram. It was hard to believe, but there he was. I can still see his face in my memory. I recall thinking, "Wow, so I can come out of this alive!" I also remember the joy that brought to my mother. She told everyone about the young man that had survived "Belsie's treatment." She still remembers the event with gratitude. It brought us so much hope and with hope comes strength.

Take a Deep Breath and Speak Normally

The fear and pain are real, but please remember, most patients prefer you neither over-dramatize the situation nor pretend everything is peachy. It is a difficult balance, but if you stay calm and focus on your friend who is battling for her life, you will be fine.

Do express your love and concern, but don't lose track of the human being in front of you. Don't let the machines and the IVs and the incessant traffic of doctors, nurses and attendants distract you. It can be disorienting to make a hospital visit if a hospital is not your natural habitat. Do your best to filter your surroundings out, assess your friend's mood, and speak as you would normally speak to her.

If you're the kind of friend who is always cracking jokes, watch your timing, but crack away.

If you share a love of books or movies and you're always discussing the latest one, go ahead and do that.

If the two of you enjoy analyzing current affairs, jump right in.

If you're both convinced that space aliens built the pyramids, share the latest theories.

You get the picture: be yourself. Protect and defend your relationship. That is one of the best things you can do for your loved one who is sick.

By being their silly, funny, intellectual and loving selves, my friends showed me why life was worth living. They brought back to my life the sense of familiar normalcy by being themselves and treating me as the same Belsie they had always known.

When you are going through intense treatment you lose control over everything, even how you look, which is part of your identity. Your routines are governed by treatment schedules and the inopportune side-effects. Having friends that acknowledged and respected the process and my fears, but behaved with me as they always had, was the best gift. They made it possible for me to enjoy each and every one of them in their uniqueness as I had before I was sick. They reminded me of one of the best parts of life: kind, loving and fun relationships.

Questions

Of course you have questions. Your friend or loved one is sick. You want to know what's going on, what is going to happen, and how you fit into this new landscape. Some of the questions my friends and family asked me were:

- What kind of cancer is it?
- How does this cancer affect your body?
- Does it hurt?
- What's the treatment?
- How long will you have to be in treatment?
- What does bone marrow do, anyway?
- What are T-cells?
- What do the doctors say?

This last question was a roundabout way of asking what everyone was wondering but no one dared to ask: *Are you going to die?*

There is nothing wrong about wanting the answer to these and other questions. The important thing is to put yourself in your friend's place. Consider the following:

- Many people will be asking the same questions.
- The patient is not sleeping well.
- The patient is under stress.

- The patient is anxious, facing the possibility of dying.
- The patient is confused about medical terms at the start of her treatment.
- The patient may not yet understand her treatment options.

For these and other reasons, the patient may not want to talk about her illness or treatment. She may prefer to enjoy the pleasure of your company and talk about other things. With this in mind, look at these options:

- The patient will have a core team of friends and family. Direct your questions to one of them instead of asking the patient.
- If you are part of this inner circle of friends and family, ask the other members and/or ...
- Do a little reading on your own to understand the basics of your friend's condition and treatment.
- If you are part of the inner circle, ask the doctors or nurses.

If you have a deeply close relationship and discuss these matters with the patient, keep the following in mind:

- Be respectful of her possible reluctance to go into details.
- Be careful about your emotional reactions to the information you receive. She is likely in a fragile emotional state. An expression of fear in your face can affect her.
- Be prudent with what you say when she shares her illness and treatment. Before you launch a tirade against corporate medicine and big pharma, find out the patient's views on the subject.

- Refer to The Iron Rule, no horror stories.

"If There is Anything I Can Do ..."

When our friend Rubén says good-by to friends, he says "Remember, if you ever need anything ... figure it out for yourself."

He's being funny, but his little joke has a point about half-hearted offers of help. This is one of the most common mistakes people make. When we say things like "Let me know if there is anything I can do," the result is usually that nothing happens. This is because most of us are reluctant to ask for help. You may feel that your friend's reluctance is not your fault. You are being sincere in your offer and if the other person has a problem asking for help that's her business. The truth is that if you offer to help with those words, you almost make sure that you will never have to do a thing. If you are sincere in your wish to help, you need to be more specific.

Ask

One way to do this is by asking how you can help. This allows your loved one to think about her needs and how you may be able to contribute. She may ask you to water her plants. She may ask you to help her set up a fundraising page online or she may ask you to do something else, depending on your relationship. Then you can say, "Yes, I can," or "I can do that, but within these parameters," or "I am allergic to cats, but I will be happy to pick up your mail."

Volunteer

Another way is to make the suggestion yourself: "I can walk your dog ... Look after the children while you go to the doctor ... Wash your car... Prepare meals ... Would that help?"

Saying "If there is anything I can do ..." is vague.

If you want to help, help. Be specific, think about your unique talents, resources and relationships and figure out how.

A Word of Advice About Advice

When someone we love is sick, we want to help.
Sometimes our desire to help leads us to offer advice we have
not studied well ourselves. It is a desperate situation. We
may feel that we should offer all options, no matter how
unorthodox. Keep in mind that your friend and her support
group are likely to have their hands full. They are dealing
with symptoms, treatment and medical directions, logistics
and finances. Throwing out suggestions about miracle
treatments or raling against the medical establishment can
sow confusion and anxiety.

If you are intrigued about alternative treatments or have
nutritional suggestions to make, do your friend a favor.
Research these ideas in more depth before presenting them.
Many people are willing to try nutritional changes and other
remedies as long as they do not interfere with their standard
treatment. If you take the time to investigate and make a
presentation, your friend may be more likely to consider
your advice.

Resist the impulse to give advice unless you are certain it
is useful. Look inside your heart. The ego can be tricky.
Remember, it's not about you. It's about your friend.

One of my mother's sisters is a vegetarian with a vast
knowledge of the benefits of fruits and vegetable. She told
my mother that carrot juice was good to boost my body's

defenses and that was all it took for my mother to make me gallons of fresh carrot juice every week. She was in warrior mode and she was going to find a way to give me anything that would seem to help. I was very receptive. If it was not going to interfere with treatment, I was going to try it. I ended up drinking so much carrot juice that my skin developed a perfect orange glow. It reminded me of how in my teens I would use an orange color suntan lotion to acquire that same glow. If I had only known then about this extra benefit of carrot juice, it would've saved me from roasting myself under the sun.

Not everyone is equally open to things out of their comfort zone. Follow their lead. You offer. If she is not receptive, let go of your expectations. You are more to her than a miracle remedy whisperer. I know you want her to heal and you believe you have the cure or something that would help, but it is her body, her journey, her choice.

"Do not let any unwholesome talk come out of your mouths, but only what is helpful for building others up according to their needs, that it may benefit those who listen."

Ephesians 4:29

Things People Say

It has happened to all of us. We mean well, but once we open our mouths in sensitive situations our nerves get the best of us. We say the wrong thing. At times we don't even notice. Those are the worst times. Other times it is like we can see our words coming out of our mouth, but it is too late. We said the words and we can't believe we did.

In the following pages you will find some common examples of things people say and the unfortunate effects these seemingly harmless words can have. But I won't leave it there. I will also share positive alternatives to express empathy and support.

Why do we so often say the wrong thing? The most common cause is fear. Fear of suffering, fear of death, fear—ironically—of saying the wrong thing. One way to deal with this fear is to acknowledge it. Look inside yourself and accept that this situation strikes fear into your heart. Why wouldn't it? Then sit with your fear and accept it without shame. It is normal. We are all afraid of dying or losing someone we love. Open your heart and open your mind to better ways. Pray for guidance. Think about a very difficult time in your life. Think about what people said to you. Think about what helped and what did not help.

If you find that you have been guilty of saying one or more of the things listed here, don't feel too bad. You're in good company. Do read the following sections, though, and take these ideas to heart. A little reflection can go a long way towards helping you become more supportive when your friend is sick.

Then go, and sin no more.

It's Nothing

There is a gap between the detection of symptoms and a definitive diagnosis. During this gap, many well-meaning friends and relatives say, "It's probably nothing." They offer anecdotes about themselves or others who had similar symptoms and found they had nothing serious.

You might think that you are trying to reassure this person you care about. What is taking place is that you are letting your fear of losing her win. Your fear is natural, but instead of dismissing the reality your friend may be facing, get suppot for your fear from others. That way, you can focus on being present and empathic for your friend.

Denial in no way supports your loved one. Pretending that it is nothing, or not that bad, only sends the message that you don't understand how she feels. That will make her feel alone.

Listening and asking questions that will give her the opportunity to talk about how she feels will allow her to express her fears. This way, you can let her know that you are there for her.

Don't think that you need to fix the situation or take the pain away. What will relieve the pain is feeling understood and unconditionally loved.

Keep in mind that it's one thing to be positive and another thing to downplay what your loved one is going through.

Everything is Going to Be Fine

Yes, that is your wish and there is power in words.
However, even the doctor treating her does not know exactly
what the outcome is going to be. Medicine is a probabilities
game. There are too many factors affecting how things are
going to turn out.

Phrases like "everything is going to be fine" come across
as empty, simplistic statements. Your friend may feel that
you are dismissing her feelings, not that you are being
positive and supportive.

By saying phrases like, "I am praying for you" or "I hope
all turns out well" you are acknowledging that the situation is
difficult, but you are staying positive. That invites the other
person to be positive as well. But you offer your support
without ignoring her feelings and by modeling how not to let
fear take over.

Asking about her thoughts gives her the opportunity to
express them and not let them build up inside. This
repression can create anxiety. It can make her feel lonely.

Something else that may be useful is to guide her back to
the present once she has expressed how she feels. For
example, if she has not received results from laboratory tests
yet, ask her, "What if we place the thoughts about the tests in

a drawer and pick them up later?" Then make the effort to change the subject. Invite her to do something. Tell her about a movie you saw or a book you have read and ask her opinion about the ideas or stories you shared. Ask her to a ball game, a movie, or to go shopping or to visit a mutual friend. Talk about what is around you, not the tests or her fears. The idea is to help her live in the present and enjoy the life that she does have.

You'll Be Out of Here in No Time

Those facing life-threatening illnesses would do well to avoid excessive optimism as much as excessive pessimism. An insight from Dr. Viktor Frankl tells us why.

Frankl, author of *Man's Search for Meaning*, noticed a pattern during his internment in German concentration camps. Those prisoners who arrived at the camps convinced that the Allies would soon come to liberate them were soon disappointed. They then fell into despair and lost the will to live. On the whole, their life expectancy in the camps was short. On the other side of the spectrum were those who gave up right away. Those, too, had short life expectancies. Then there was the third group. Those prisoners who accepted that they would be prisoners for a long time, but who at the same time kept believing that they would eventually be free, adjusted better. They tended to live longer.

Dr. Flankl's insights are relevant to those facing life-threatening illnesses. It may be better to seek a balance. It may be better to accept that treatment will take time. It may be better to accept that it will bring hardships and that a happy outcome is not guaranteed. Better to do this while they also take one day at a time and look for small reasons to find solace.

The same is true for friends and family of the person facing the illness.

Expressions of excessive optimism may rub your friend the wrong way. She is aware of the seriousness of her situation. She may take your expressions as dismissive of her pain and fear. Furthermore, the disappointment that is likely to follow such excessive optimism will be evident at some point. This will become an additional emotional burden for your friend. This is the last thing she needs. Take the middle way.

Don't Cry

Sadness is a natural reaction when your friend is facing a threat to her life. If you fail to acknowledge this, your friend may feel that you don't understand what she is going through. She may retreat into herself, losing hope that anyone will understand her feelings. There is no worse illness that loneliness.

We often have the misguided impression that by saying things like "don't be sad" or "don't cry" we will help make the pain go away. You might feel better if your loved one stops crying, but this only imposes another burden on her: now she has to take care of *your* feelings. In the end, neither your pain nor your loved one's pain will go away with those phrases. However, silence and gentle gestures will help her feel your love and will comfort her heart.

Asking about her feelings will give her the opportunity to process her pain. Let her guide you. If you see that she is not responding, let her be. She might not be ready yet. Your interest is not going to offend her, but do not insist. Give her some time and ask again later.

Have You Vomited Today?

There are personal matters that we prefer not to remember or that we don't care to discuss with others. Unless your friend mentions them, don't bring those up. Trust me, we will mention them when we need to talk about them. Most likely we will enjoy talking about anything else. We are with our symptoms and treatment all day long. Although we need venting sessions occasionally, let your friend choose the time and the reason. In the meantime, other topics are welcome!

Wow! You've Lost a Lot of Weight!

Gee ... thanks?

Your friend knows she has lost weight.

If you have information about supplemental smoothies or juices, feel free to offer them, but know that some will not like those suggestions. You might want to tell a family member instead of going to the person who is sick or recovering.

I welcomed anything natural or proven to provide nutrients. My treatment affected my appetite and ravaged my digestive system. I welcomed anything that would help me get nutrients without upsetting my stomach. Juices and prepared shakes I bought in drugstores and supermarkets were better for me than full meals. I remember how for periods of time those were the only things I could ingest. I had to drink them slowly to make sure they would not upset my stomach. My mother told me, "Drink them as if they are medicine," and that did the trick. I had started my treatment saying, "If I am going to go through this treatment, I am going play to win." This is why I saw smoothies and shakes and dietary changes as tools to help me accomplish that goal.

Comments about how much weight your friend has lost are not helpful. Supporting your friend in celebrating what works for her is.

Have You Thought of Wearing a Wig?

During my illness, my brother became some sort of guardian angel and CEO of my life. He had been living abroad and had returned home to look out for me and my Mom. He helped coordinate everything related to my treatment. One day he was wearing his handyman hat. He was fixing some things around the house and needed to go pick up supplies. I heard him open the car door and I went outside. I asked him where he was going. Having him around made me feel safe and he was great company. He invited me to go with him so I would get out of the house and get a change of scenery.

"Wait," I said, "let me go get something to cover my head."

I was bald by then and although I never wore a wig, I did wear scarfs and hats.

"You are fine that way," he said. "Come with me."

I smiled and got in the car and off we went. I remember lowering the visor to look at myself in the mirror.

"You look beautiful," he said.

"People are going to be looking at me as if I am from another planet," I said.

I had never seen any bald women walking around in our little town or anywhere else.

"It is a matter of attitude," he said. "If you walk with your head up, feeling beautiful, people will only see a beautiful woman."

He is one of my older brothers. All he says has always had a great impact on me. I walked tall by his side (at my full five-foot-zero) and realized no one was staring at me the way I thought they would. I remember smiling big and looking at him as if to say, "You were right."

He smiled. His smile said, "I am proud of you."

That was when I started to feel beautiful. I had never felt pretty growing up. Chemotherapy got rid of cancer—and some insecurities as well!

Physical appearance is important to both men and women, so if you can't help by saying something complimentary, it's better to say nothing at all. Respect your friend's wishes and let her lead the way. Whether she chooses to cover her head or wear makeup, dress up or down, always focus on the positive. Never focus on the negative.

You Need to Get Out of the House

Depending on the severity of the treatment, we have little control over our lives. Our schedules are now filled medical appointments. The side effects drain our energy for daily chores. We don't even look the way we used to. We will receive your suggestions about what we should or shouldn't do if you talk to us as if we were your healthy colleague or friend. When we are healthy our friends invite us to do things with them. They don't give us orders or lectures.

When thinking about what to say or do, think about normalcy. There is nothing we want more than feeling that we've got our lives back. We want to life to feel the way it did before we were sick. We want to go back to when we did not have to worry about fighting for our lives. We still remember when we could eat what we wanted. We want to feel as we did when we could look to our future without fear of never getting there.

If you feel your friend should get out more, invite her out.

I'm Having Such a Bad Day!

Really?

It is true that honesty is the best policy in any relationship, but let's put things in perspective. Your friend or family member is fighting for her life. Unless you are at the same time fighting for your life, it is very unlikely that your day is going to compare to hers.

Go ahead and talk about your day, but remember in whose company you are. If you focus too much on what it is negative in your life, you will miss the opportunity to hear what it is going on her life. In fact, being with someone who is fighting for her life is a reminder of something important. In spite of your own troubles, you are in fact lucky not to be on the other side. Count your blessings, and share those.

Say THIS, Not THAT

Say:	Not:
What is your main concern?	It is probably nothing. I had a headache (infection, mass, pain...) and it turned out to be nothing. My aunt once had the same symptoms and it turned out to be nothing.
I cannot know how you feel, but I can imagine that this is intimidating. Know that I am here for you. You can count on my prayers, well wishes ... What is on your mind right now? Based on her comfort: Hold her hand, put your arm around her. Hold her. I am sorry you are having to go through this. Know that I am here for you.	Don't be sad. Don't cry.
Have you received the	Everything is going to be OK.

results of your laboratory test results? What did the doctor say? How do you feel about what the doctor said? Would you like me to pray with you? I will pray for everything to turn out well.	You are not going to die.
How is your appetite?	Have you vomited today?
I heard of this new place! If you feel like it, I would like you to come with me. My treat! I remembered how much you like eating [a type of food or at a restaurant]. Let's go together. I am craving [some kind of food] would you like to go with me?	You are disappearing. You look skinny. You have lost a lot of weight.

I am concerned about your weight loss. How is your appetite?	
Your head has the best shape! Now your eyes stand out more. You have a beautiful smile!	Have you thought about wearing a wig? You look pale.
I could use a walk; would you go with me? I need to run some errands and I don't want to do them by myself. Would you go with me? I was thinking about going back to that park/mall/festival and who better to go with than you?	You need to get out of this house.
Spending time with you will make my day better.	I am having such a bad day!

It has not been my best day, but I am glad to be talking with you. How is yours going?	
Tell stories about positive events, beautiful places or funny memories. Or best yet—make plans!	I just learned that the mother of a neighbor died after having something similar.

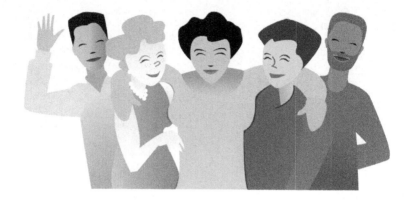

"When you do things from your soul, you feel a river moving in you, a joy."

— Rumi

WHAT TO DO

So far we have discussed what to say when a friend is sick. Now we are going to examine the things people do. We will discuss what I and others found helpful and not so helpful during treatment or recovery. Some of these examples will touch back upon some of the topics in the previous sections.

In those sections we have looked at how, despite our good intentions, our fears and lead us to say things that are not constructive. In some cases, our words can have negative consequences for the very friend we wish to help. The same holds true of the things we do—or don't do—in these cases. With a little less haste and a little more thought we can turn those good intentions into good actions. Ready? Let's go.

"Everybody can be great ... because anybody can serve. You don't have to have a college degree to serve. You don't have to make your subject and verb agree to serve. You only need a heart full of grace. A soul generated by love."

— Dr. Martin Luther King, Jr.

The Amazing Vanishing Friend Act

One of the things that disconcerted me the most was when one of my friends disappeared after my diagnosis. He was close friend; we were in frequent contact and I knew he was aware of my illness. Nevertheless, he never visited me in the hospital, he never called, he didn't even send a card. He pulled the Amazing Vanishing Friend Act. At first I was sad and disappointed because I expected more of him. As time went by, however, I not only felt sad because of missing him, but I also felt sad for him. I felt sad because I understood that he was afraid. I also felt sad because his fear of doing or saying the wrong thing was stronger than his friendship.

Don't allow your awkwardness and fear to turn you into the Amazing Vanishing Friend. It is my hope that by now you have a better idea about what to say and what not to say. When it comes to what to do, the very first thing to keep in mind is this: be there.

Everything else comes later. If you go to the hospital, do so. If you can visit at home, visit at home. If you're too far away to visit in person, pick up the phone. Send an email message. Send a text message. If your friend is not well enough to reply, chances are someone else in her inner circle is checking her messages. At least your friend will know that you made an effort.

Whether you hear back from your friend or someone in her team, follow up. Again, you don't have to be a great writer. The fact is that after the novelty of the diagnosis wears off, people tend to drop out of view. Your friend can get lonely in her hospital room—and even in her home— when she's sick for a long time. Hearing from you from time to time, even if you send a short message, means more than you know.

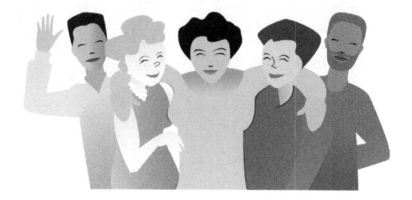

"For it is in giving that we receive".

-St. Francis of Assisi

You Do You (Be-Do-Be-Do)

One of my closest friends came to visit me. She said hello the way she usually did. She started our conversation the way we always did. We talked about mutual friends and we updated each other on the latest who did what and who said what to whom. We looked at some catalogs and talked about fashion: what we liked, what we didn't like. We joked and laughed and drank some fruit juice and talked some more. We looked at more catalogs. Then the sun went down, the breeze grew cooler and we said our good-byes.

When my friend went home, she spoke to her mother on the phone.

"How's Belsie?" Her mother asked.

"She's fine," my friend said.

"How's her condition?"

"I don't know."

"What do the doctors say?"

"I don't know."

"What do you mean, you don't know?"

91

"It means I don't know."

"Didn't you say you just saw her?"

"I just saw her, yes."

"Then how can you not know?"

"We didn't talk about it."

"Then what did you talk about?"

"I don't know ... life."

There you have it. We talked about life. My friend, God bless her, did a wonderful thing: she was herself. She treated me, not as a cancer patient, but as her lifelong friend. She didn't focus on my illness or my symptoms. She focused on me. By being the same as she had always been, she allowed me to be the way I had always been before falling down the rabbit hole of my illness. This is one of the many reasons I love her.

Whoever you are in your friend's life, be that person. Do what you do. Yes, there may be some things your friend cannot do while she is ill. She may be facing some limitations. She may get tired quickly. She may have to stay out of the sun. Many things may be different now, but as far as you are able, be that special someone you are in your friend's life.

You don't have to talk about the illness all the time. You don't have to try to cheer her up all the time. If you're the friend who always has a joke ready, be that friend. If you're the friend who looks for new recipes to share, be that friend. If you're the friend who provides political analysis, be that friend. Remember, you play a role in your friend's life that nobody else can play.

R.E.S.P.E.C.T. Your Friend's Wishes

You may have some ideas about what is good for your sick friend. As always, your intentions are good. You want to see your friend healthy again. You want to see her happy. Only, your friend may have different views. She wants to be well and happy too, but she may not agree with you on every step she needs to take to get there. If you have a difference of opinion, respect your friend's wishes. As long as she is not endangering herself, let her lead the way.

This applies to all sorts of things.

If you feel she should get out of the house and she prefers to stay home, respect her wishes. She may not have the physical energy to go out.

If you feel she should try that new smoothie you discovered but she begs off, respect her wishes. You can leave her the recipe. Treatment sometimes affects the way things taste. What tastes wonderful to you may taste like cardboard to her. She may circle back to your smoothie later.

If she prefers to wear a wig to cover her head and you think she should go bald, respect her wishes. Mention you think she has a well-shaped head and leave it at that. Some people need a little time to adjust to their new look. Others never do.

If she prefers to cover her head with brightly colored scarves or men's hats and you think she should wear a wig, stop and think. Is she enjoying her scarves? Is she collecting different kinds of hats? Respect her wishes. With a bit of luck she'll get her hair back soon enough. In the meantime, let her have some fun with her headdress.

If she decides this is the perfect time to go vegan, as long as she's getting the nutrition she needs, respect her wishes. You may have no desire to go vegan, but your friend has not become less able to make her own decisions because she is sick. Who knows? You may come to like vegan food.

Step Up: Volunteer

My good friend, Mari, used to come to visit every single day. This one Saturday, she was surprised to find my room dark: no lights, no open windows. That was unusual. My mom would always make sure there was natural light coming in the room. She believed that sunlight was helpful in improving my mood.

"Why so dark?" Mari asked. I told her I had woken up with conjunctivitis and the light was bothering me. She expressed empathy and continued talking a bit more. After a while, she excused herself and said she would come back. About 30 minutes later, she returned. She was carrying a pair of clip-on sunglasses that fit over my glasses and *voilà* – let there be light! We were able to open the windows and let the sunlight back in! This was also helpful for my mother, who was by my side day in and day out.

No one had asked Mari to do anything—neither my mother nor I had complained about the dark room. Mari noticed and took it upon herself to find a remedy.

If you see a similar opportunity to do something that will be helpful, go ahead and do it. If what you propose to do is not quite as straightforward, ask if your friend would mind if you carried out your plan. Remember the old "If there is anything I can do ..." principle. Volunteer to do something specific.

All Together Now!

A group of former classmates and I were coordinating our 10th high school class reunion when I received my second leukemia diagnosis. We had made plenty of progress and were looking forward to the great day, but I had to leave town to receive treatment. It was quite a disappointment for me. I remember wondering on the day of the party who had come and how things were going.

Days later, my friend Lourdes showed up at the hospital. She had with her a gigantic card, 3 feet tall. It had illustrations she had drawn herself and messages from my classmates. She had passed the card around for all to sign. Lourdes is a kind and very talented woman who takes advantage of any opportunity to give. She also filmed greetings from my classmates. They expressed their love and sent get well wishes. Reading the messages in the card and watching the video was the best gift! It warmed my heart. There is no doubt that love heals. The joy in their voices and their warm messages gave me new energy to continue with the treatment. The joint effort and their words reminded me of the beauty of connection, sharing and loving. I would have never even thought of such creative ways to bring joy to someone's heart.

Observe, listen and let your heart lead you. You will not need great sums of money or great lengths of time. Put your talents at the service of those you love. You might only be able to draw stick figures. Your filming abilities may make people dizzy. But you might be able to take pictures of beautiful places, cook, or drive to the supermarket or give a dog a bath. Everything counts, believe me! Every gesture supports healing.

You Got Mail!

Before my diagnosis, I met Manolo when he came from Spain to visit his family in Puerto Rico. He went back to Spain and months passed. I did not hear from him again. When his family told him I was sick, he started writing me letters.

Yes, letters. On paper. By mail. Not email, not text messages, not social media. Letters. His letters came in distinctive envelopes with a red and blue printed border. Every time the mail would arrive, I would glance at the pack of letters and know if there was one from him.

The letters were friendly ones that would transport me to another world. He also sent me books about different subjects. He would send philosophy books and poetry books. Manolo was in a different continent, thousands of miles away. He was even in a different time zone, but he gave me something to look forward to.

Even today, there is something special about receiving a real letter. Try writing letters to your sick friend. Put pen to paper. Choose a cheerful or beautiful card or some good paper stock. Select a special postage stamp. You don't have to be a famous letter writer like Emily Dickinson or Flannery O'Connor to write great letters. You just need to be a friend.

Hospital Visits

Hospitals are no fun. Nurses are constantly poking you, sticking you with needles and waking you up. Plus there's the whole facing-a-life-threatening-illness thing. For all these reasons, we do love to welcome our dear friends when they visit but sometimes we are too tired or too ill to receive visits. This is why it is always a good idea to call ahead and ask whether your friend is able to see you.

Visiting your friend, however, is not the only reason to go to the hospital. As we said earlier, caregivers need support, too. Your visit may be the one chance your friend's caregivers have to take a walk, catch a movie or get a massage. You may find that you spend your visit chatting with a caregiver while your friend sleeps. This gives the caregiver a welcome change of pace. You may discover during your visit that your friend needs a new set of pajamas and decide to go get them.

There are many reasons to visit at the hospital. Just remember a few things.

• If your friend is in a shared room, be considerate of the other patient.

• Even if your friend is in a private room, be mindful of how much space is available. If there are too many people in the room, go in the hallway for a while. Get some fresh air. Don't crowd your friend.

• Mind your volume. It's wonderful to laugh with your friend, but remember there are other patients nearby.

• During some stages of treatment, your friend's immune system may be weak. Don't visit if you're not feeling well. If you have a cold, stay home.

• Respect the rules: if you're asked to wear a mask, wear it. If you're not comfortable with a mask, excuse yourself and plan to visit some other time.

• Always wash your hands, even if you are not planning to touch the patient.

• Remember The Iron Rule: no horror stories.

Home Visits

With a little luck, your friend will be back home before too long. She will continue her treatment at home or rest while she gets better. It's easy to imagine that once your friend is out of the hospital, she's fine. This is not necessarily the case. She may have challenging symptoms or side effects from her treatment. Furthermore, it is easy to become isolated while being sick at home.

During my illness I had to stop working, so I gave up my apartment. Fortunately, my mother welcomed me back home. One of my favorite things when I was home between chemo sessions was welcoming my friends at my mother's house.

• Visiting your friend at home gives you many opportunities to help.

• You can watch movies together.

• You can listen to music and even dance.

• You can bring food that was not allowed at the hospital.

• You can play table games.

• You can see whether your friend needs help with housekeeping.

• You can help with her laundry.

• You can iron a few things.

• You can take her dog for a walk.

• You can change the kitty litter.

• You can water her plants.

• You can pick up her laundry.

• You can read to her.

You can do all this and more, always keeping in mind that the best thing you can do is to continue being the friend you have been up to now. If your friend lives with her spouse and/or children, you can give them a chance to go out by themselves while you visit.

Don't expect your friend to wait on you. You are a guest in your friend's home, but you don't want to give her extra work during your visit. If there is anything you need (a glass of water, for example), ask if you can help yourself.

Also, keep track of time. Your friend may not feel comfortable telling you she needs to rest. She doesn't want to feel she's kicking you out of the house. Remember she doesn't have her usual level of energy. Know when it's time to go. If your friend falls asleep in the middle of your conversation, leave quietly.

Finances

In our western culture, most of us feel uncomfortable talking about money. Yet the fact remains that, especially in the United States, healthcare costs are outrageous. Facing a serious illness can present families with great challenges. Add to the medical costs the fact that the patient's productivity during her illness may go down to zero, and the family faces a double threat. What can you do to help in such a situation?

Everything Counts

First, remember that every little bit counts. If you are able to offer significant financial support, by all means do so. If you aren't, there is still plenty you can do. Don't dismiss your ability to help because you are not able to write a big check. You can help your friend save by cooking meals. You can help with housekeeping and home repairs and many other things.

Giving

Whether you plan to offer cash or help, though, remember that a true gift has no strings. If you give, open your heart as well as your hand. Give your gift and give up your desire to control how your friend spends her money. Yes, even if you gave her that money, it belongs to her now.

Make your peace with that fact. If you feel you have a right to say how your friend invests her resources, think again. If you can't give up your need to control, you are giving to get. That's not a gift. That's a transaction.

Lending

Be careful with lending. If your friend is facing a life-threatening illness, there is a chance she may not be able to pay you back. Can you afford to say good-bye to that money? The old saying advices that to keep your friends, "neither a borrower nor a lender be." At no time is this more true than when your friend's life is in the balance.

Be Gentle

Remember that most people are uncomfortable when they talk about money. Be tactful in your approach, especially if you are not a part of your friend's inner circle.

Kitchen Duty

After heavy chemotherapy my white cell count crashed. I had no energy, my appetite had vanished, and even food commercials on TV would make me sick. Raquel was a friend of my aunt's. I had never met her before my illness. She took it upon herself to be a guardian angel to my mother and me. She was an unassuming, intelligent, elegant lady. She had a gentle demeanor, but she was committed to always being of service. Raquel was also a strong advocate for us at the hospital and a relentless supporter.

One day she came to visit but, instead of showing up at the hospital like she usually did, she called first. She asked how my tummy was feeling. It was the perfect day to ask that question. I was feeling much better and could use a good non-hospital meal. She asked me if I had a craving for something in particular. I told her about this pasta dish that I would eat from a chain restaurant back home. Raquel decided to find this dish. She went to restaurant after restaurant all over town. Time after time she struck out, until at last she found something very similar.

The gesture meant so much to me that I still remember it more than 20 years later. Raquel knew how important it was for me to eat. She thought, "If she is feeling better, putting something enticing in front of her might stimulate her appetite. That way, she'll get some calories." She accomplished both goals. Those were the days when I was not concerned about gaining weight!

Raquel had been paying attention. She figured that a warm, tasty meal was something she could offer to support my recovery process. No one asked her to go around the city looking for the dish I was craving. She was not even my aunt. She had not even met me before I got sick. She let compassion lead her way and I am eternally grateful.

If you can follow Raquel's lead, by all means do so. Even one meal is important. You can also organize a group of friends to take turns preparing meals, or even the occasional cake!

Your friend will thank you.

Clean Up Day

Chemotherapy and other treatments weaken our immune system. This leaves us vulnerable to all kinds of diseases. That is why it's so important to keep our environment clean. Germs and allergens can affect patients more than other people. When you visit the hospital, doctors may ask you to wear a mask. The mask blocks any germs you may be carrying. Germs can travel in micro-drops of saliva, which can travel up to six feet in front of you when you speak.

Going home after a prolonged absence requires a thorough cleanup day. If your friend does not have domestic help, it may fall to others to do this job. Her spouse, family or friends must ensure that her environment is clean for her return home. Once she has settled in, the place needs to stay clean. Chances are your friend will not be able to help with that work for some time.

Helping in this area may mean paying for someone to do the work. You can pay yourself or with the help of other friends. It may also mean doing the work yourself or taking turns with others. Whatever you are able to do, it is important to remember that a clean space is important for a person facing a life-threatening illness. This is true not only for physical health reasons. A clean and organized space is also bound to help your friend's state of mind. This will allow her to concentrate on what ought to be her only job at the moment: getting well.

Road Trip!

I sometimes alternated between chemo sessions and all-nighters at the emergency room. This was when my platelets crashed. On good days, we would take road trips. At the time, I was living in Puerto Rico, a tropical island. There was beautiful weather most of the time and there were plenty of lovely places to visit. As long as we had clear skies and I was feeling well enough, the gang and I would climb in a car and hit the road. The gang was usually my brother and a few of my friends. At other times we would look at the map of the island and read magazines to plan future excursions. I learned a good deal about my island home in those days. I also had wonderful times that made me forget I was fighting for my life. I will always remember them.

I know what you're thinking: "That's great for you, Belsie, but I don't live in some beautiful island paradise." I understand. Not everyone lives in Puerto Rico, or in Hawaii, or in Key West. Whether you are in Marco Island or Fargo, there are places near you that you have been meaning to visit. Look for botanical gardens, state or national parks or places of historical importance, like St. Augustine, Florida or the Jefferson Memorial. What about Mt. Rushmore, or the Grand Canyon? The world is full of beautiful, inspiring places. Go as soon as the weather allows.

You can take a day trip. You can even stay overnight. This is the sort of thing that is always available to us, but we find reasons to put them off. For my family, my friends and me, it took the prospect of never seeing these places to get us on the road. Once we started, the idea stuck. Now we make sure to take road trips to explore new places whenever we can.

Where will you go on your next road trip? Where will you help your friend create great new memories? It's a big, beautiful world out there. You don't need a lot to go. All you need is a car and a wandering spirit.

Pick a destination. Hit the road!

Religion and Spirituality

When facing life-and-death situations, most of us turn to our religious and spiritual beliefs. We seek comfort in the middle of the pain and uncertainty. Since we find comfort in our beliefs, we want to offer that comfort to our ailing friend. Thus, we want to talk to our friend about those beliefs. So far, so good.

If you know that your friend is receptive to your views—if you know each other from church, for example—then it's smooth sailing for you. If you are not familiar with her views, or if you don't know if she will welcome your input , tread lightly. Go back to the Live Your Values section.

If you want to pray for your friend in her hospital room, ask her if she feels comfortable with this. Respect her wishes. You can always pray at home. If you share literature with your friend, be gentle when you ask if she has had a chance to read it. She sort of has a full-time job right now: getting better. Don't push her. You may feel it's urgent for her to receive what you're offering her. Be patient. Have faith.

This also applies, by the way, if you happen to be an atheist or agnostic. Your friend is fighting for her life, or handling the effects of a serious illness. Religion may or may not be the opiate of the people, but your friend may well be taking real opiates to relieve her pain. This is not the time to engage in philosophical debates. There are many other topics of conversation. There are other things you can do to help your friend feel better. Be compassionate, be kind. You can have those debates later.

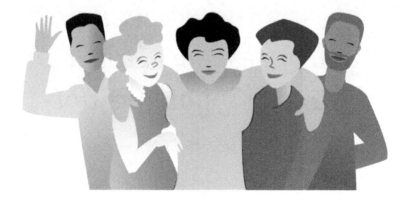

"When you love someone, the best thing you can offer is your presence. How can you love if you are not there?"

— Thich Nhat Hanh

WHAT TO GIVE

We have discussed what to say and what to do when a friend is sick. In looking at what to do, we have touched upon the idea of offering different things to our sick friend or her family. Now we'll take a closer look at what to give.

It is important, when offering any kind of gift, to be mindful of what the person receiving the gift wants and needs. This is not always obvious. Too often we offer what we think the person needs without taking the time to ask or find out. That's when our gift gets a lukewarm reception. We already mentioned the importance of asking specific questions when volunteering any sort of help. If we feel the desire to offer a gift, asking questions is important. You can ask your friend or you can ask her close friends or family. What does she need right now?

When we speak of gifts we don't only mean material gifts, like a comfortable pillow or a luxurious robe—or a luxury Italian sports car. These are welcome, but there are many other kinds of gifts we can offer. The important thing is to match the gift to the recipient, and to do that we need to step outside ourselves and what we imagine we would want in our friend's situation. Instead, explore what would truly be appreciated.

Oh, and remember, a true gift has no strings.

The Languages of Love

In his wonderful book, *The 5 Love Languages: The Secret to Love That Lasts*, Gary Chapman explains there are different ways in which we give and receive love. These are our love languages. Each of us has a primary love language. Though we may speak the other languages, this is the main way we communicate our affection. To improve our chances of developing healthy and enduring relationships, it is helpful to identify our own love language. It is also key to identify the other person's love language.

The five love languages Chapman discusses in his book are:

1. Words of Affirmation

2. Quality Time

3. Receiving Gifts

4. Acts of Service

5. Physical Touch

Chapman is a marriage counselor and he wrote his book mainly for couples. However, his insights are useful for all kinds of relationships. Pick it up and see if you can determine your sick friend's love language. The author speaks in a friendly and accessible style. He uses many anecdotes that illustrate his ideas and it's a quick read. Be sure to read the section on Discovering Your Primary Love Language.

The Gift of Spirituality

My oldest brother and his wife are strong Christians.
They live and breathe their faith. However, not once did they
try to convert me or force their spiritual beliefs on me. They
would come to visit and mention verses from the Bible that
would reinforce their belief that God was watching after me
and that He wanted to and could heal me, but they never
said that if I didn't accept this as the sole truth I would die. I
am inquisitive by nature, so I would ask them about various
aspects of faith and they would gently explain and guide me
to find my own answers. It was a positive experience that
changed my life and allowed me to develop the solid faith I
have now.

One day we finally convinced my mother not to spend
the night at the hospital. The first time my mother had spent
the night away from me I had had a severe reaction to
treatment. Since then, she had refused to leave my bedside.
My sister-in-law was the designated companion for this
night. I was looking forward to her stay. She and I had been
very close when I was little. And sure enough, she did not
disappoint. She entered the room singing the choir of a
Christian song that I still sing in my head when I am afraid
or nervous, "Jesus is passing through and when He comes
through everything gets transformed; sadness is gone,
happiness arrives ..." We had a great night.

If you are a believer, make sure you share to lift and not to condemn.

The Gift of Caring for the Caregiver

Sometimes the best thing you can do for someone is to take care of the people she loves. In my case it was my mother. My mother had retired after more than 30 years of working every day as a nurse to take care of four children. She had become a widow at the age of 41 and had never remarried. Instead of enjoying her well-earned retirement, she was spending day and night taking care of me in the hospital.

One day her sister Perla came to visit. After much pleading, she finally convinced my mother to leave the hospital with her. Perla is an award-winning hair stylist and she adores my mother. She knew exactly what my mother needed. She took her to the house of one of my other aunts and washed, cut and styled my mother's hair. When Perla was finished, my mother looked like herself again. Anyone who has met my mother even once, will comment on how well she carries herself. Suddenly she was smiling again and she had new stories to tell.

I was always grateful to have my mother by my side. Yet, seeing her every day sleeping in a cot or a chair at her age, after all the other sacrifices she had made for my siblings and me, was a great burden. That day my aunt thought she was taking care of my mother and giving her a break. She did that, and much more. The bonus was the joy I felt when I saw that my mother was feeling like herself again and had been able to spend time outside of the cold walls of the hospital.

Whether your friend's caregiver is a parent, a spouse or a sibling, think of how you can help that person. Relieve her at the hospital. Take her out for a makeover. Invite her to a spa or a nice dinner. It may be one of the best gifts you can give your friend.

The Gift of Practicality

Mom's friend, Doña Tere, is a great example of good intentions perfectly attuned to the needs of someone who is fighting for her life. One day Doña Tere came to visit Mom and me at the hospital carrying a medium size white paper shopping bag. Mom thanked her and put the bag aside while carrying on a conversation with her. Doña Tere would drive an hour to reach us but would only stay for a short period of time. Her gentle demeanor was a reflection of her spirituality. She is a woman of great faith, and she would exude love when she showed up.

After Doña Tere left, I remember Mom bringing the bag to me.

"This Tere, she is so kind," she said, "coming all the way here with things for us. Let's see what she brought."

The bag turned out to be full of practical items: thick white socks to keep my feet warm, rubbing alcohol, body lotions and other things. Every time we pulled one out to use it, we would send a blessing her way. The things were not pretty or expensive, nor were things that we couldn't buy, or that we asked for. She just knew they were exactly what we needed. Doña Tere was giving us small tokens of love that also were useful everyday things.

The Gift of Privacy

Remember the section titled *Have You Vomited Today?* Being ill involves many things that many people don't feel comfortable discussing.

Although our bodies all have the same essential functions—allowing for differences of gender—we like to pretend many of these functions don't exist. We will not debate whether this is good or bad. The fact remains that most of us feel uncomfortable about some of the things our bodies do. A sure way to make people uncomfortable at a cocktail party, for example, is to start talking about bodily fluids. A serious illness and its treatment can bring about diarrhea, constipation, vomiting, rashes, sores and other things we would rather not discuss.

A serious illness can also affect our sex life during treatment and even for some time after we appear to be well. This is another thing we may have trouble discussing, even with our romantic partner. Every case is different and in every case it is important to give your friend the gift of privacy. With few exceptions, it is best to let your friend lead and to respect her wishes. In the case above, for example, if you are the person's romantic partner, at some point you will want to discuss your intimate life. If she doesn't bring it up, though, let it go. In most cases things will gradually go back to normal. If you're concerned, speak to your partner about seeking professional counseling that can help both of you find each other in your intimate space again.

The Gift of Silence

As much as we appreciate company and the feeling that we are not alone in our fight, sometimes the best gift can be the gift of silence. I remember times during some of our road trips when I was glad to be with my friends and at the same time I was glad they allowed me the space to be alone with my thoughts. Looking out the car window as the beautiful landscapes of my island home rolled by or strolling through a colonial town square, the silence was a balm for my troubled soul.

Don't feel you have to fill in the silence. Short gaps in your conversation can be fine. Leave them alone. The most important thing you can do is to be present, really present, fully and unmistakably. Of course you are anxious: your friend is ill. But don't let your nerves turn you into a chatterbox. Listen.

"You can make more friends in two months by becoming genuinely interested in other people than you can in two years by trying to get other people interested in you." So wrote Dale Carnegie in his 1937 book, *How to Win Friends and Influence People*. The Gottman Institute (Seattle, WA) says, "While Carnegie's advice centers on friendship and sales, our research shows that you can apply the same principles to build better relationships with your spouse, your siblings, your children, your boss—anyone who plays a significant role in your life." They advise us to "focus on being interested, not interesting."

Look into your friend's eyes from time to time. Let her know that for that moment, while your are together, she is the most important thing in your mind. Take a ride together if you can. Walk the dog. Watch the sun set. Let the silence frame the beauty of your time together.

Or let her be. Give her the gift of silence.

The Gift of Touch

When we talk about the gift of touch, we are not speaking only about sexual touch. That is, of course, a beautiful thing within the context of a consensual relationship, but we are talking here about much more. We are talking about platonic touch: taking someone's hand, a pat on the back, a friendly hug. When we are very sick, the symptoms and the effects of treatment can leave us feeling ugly, untouchable. Even our personal scent changes because of the illness and the medications. Knowing that our loved ones are not afraid to reach out and touch us in solidarity when we may not be feeling attractive can be very encouraging.

Different cultures have different rules about physical touch. Indeed, different families feel different about this subject. Some people are huggers; others shy away from public displays of affection. When appropriate, however, physical touch can be an important mood booster. The closer you are in your relationship with this person who is fighting for her life, the more important your touch is bound to be and the better able you will be to determine if it is appropriate to reach out and touch. It can elevate her mood and strengthen her hope. This is especially true of older individuals.

Older people may have already lost a spouse. They may live by themselves. They may already be living with a deficit of the comfort offered by physical contact with other people. Keep this in mind. Within the context of your relationship, be generous with the gift of your platonic touch.

There was a period of time when I was placed in isolation. Just a small number of people had access to my room in the hospital. No one was supposed to come too close to me, to avoid any possible transmission of germs. My friend Mari would come and squeeze my big toes over the blanket covering them. She would look at me with a face full of love and make a funny face.

"Ay, Nena, Nena, Nena" she would say. *Oh, Girl, Girl, Girl.* I understood—she was hugging me. It would always make me smile.

Another dear friend, Julie, had become a stylist. As part of her training, she had learned how to give hand massages. The day she came to see me I was in better shape and the doctors allowed her to give me a hand massage. Oh my! I still remember how great it felt. It was my first ever. I had no idea a hand massage could relax you so much.

Both friends gave what they could give me at the moment and they made a great contribution to my day.

The Gift of Normal

I spent my 25th and 26th birthdays in two different hospitals. Yet my memories of those days are of the gifts and cakes my family brought me. It is all about feeling normal again, feeling that there is life outside of chemotherapy and radiation. Even for at least a moment, I was the "birthday girl" not a cancer patient. I had a cake and a wish to make as I was blowing out the candle. In the pictures I have from one of those times, I am showing off my gifts, including a fashionable hat and nice trendy leather shoes. I was bald and connected to an IV pole, but I had a big smile.

The gifts were practical. I remember that I also received a coloring book and a big box of crayons. I liked coloring before adult coloring was a thing! No hospital-focused gifts, you see. No pajamas or robes, although those were also great when I received them. These gifts talked to me about life beyond the treatments.

How can you give your friend the gift of normalcy? How can you create a little oasis to help her forget, at least for a moment, all the challenges of her condition and the uncertainty of her future?

The Gift of Home: Angels in Texas

By the time the leukemia came back, I had restarted my life. I was going to graduate school, but had to drop out and move away to receive treatment, this time in Houston, Texas. I was a broke student in her 20s with a retired mother and no back up plan.

When I arrived for my pre-treatment evaluations, my mother and I first stayed in a friend's one-bedroom apartment where she lived with her mother. This friend was Angel #1. My mother and I slept on their sofa-bed until I was admitted into the hospital. Once I was discharged, we stayed in another friend's house (Angel #2) while waiting for an apartment close to the hospital to be available. On both occasions, families had to adjust their lives and spaces to fit the two of us. My mother and I are only five feet tall. We only weigh a little over a hundred pounds each. We did not take up much space and we did everything possible not to disturb their lives. But no doubt we were at least two small impositions. Their generosity and their kindness were much more than we had hoped for.

We were finally able to rent an apartment, but again with finances running ever so thin, we needed help. Enter my third angel, Janet, an old friend of my brother's. My brother had come with us to look after my mother and me and to help us settle in Houston. By the time my mother and I moved into the new apartment, there was even dishwashing liquid in the sink. Janet had brought things from her own house to turn that apartment into a home for us—from furniture to dish towels. Everything was there. She showed my brother where to buy at discount prices the few things we had to buy. As if that was not enough, she gave us a free membership to the most important art museum in town. Janet is a talented artist and she knew the healing power of art and how nourishing our visits to the museum would be.

We had many difficult times going through treatment in Houston, but the love we received balanced it all out. Some people opened up their homes for us and others turned a regular apartment into a real home for us.

My mother always says that God places angels in our path. I have no doubt that this is true and that I have met many of them. Without my angels on earth, I would not be here to tell you these stories.

The Gift of Reading and Music

My partners in healing were a group of friends and family members who formed a team of love, support and fun around me. Any team, e.g., sports, work, faith-based, have several members and each one has a specific role. Not everyone can be the captain and the captain alone can't face an entire opposing team and still win. Further, not all members of a team are on the court at once. The same happens with healing partners. There were key players and each one had an important role at a specific time.

In a game there are also recesses. I found that recess could be risky, if I didn't know how to manage my thoughts. Recess was supposed to be for resting, but fear could take over and I could find myself falling down a spiral of dismay and hopelessness.

Here are some gifts I received that became tools to help me stay focused on the goal and not on the circumstances:

A Bible – My oldest brother gave me a beautiful Bible with a burgundy leather-soft cover with my name engraved on it. I remember the nice smell of the pages. I still have it although now it has asterisks, highlighted passages and underlined words.

When I did not have visitors, I would read psalms and chapters either my brother or friends recommended. It was a great tool to remind me of the love of God, His protection and strength in me.

Christian Music – My oldest brother also brought me cassettes of Christian music. That was such a gift. I would listen to them over and over again. By the time I had to go through scary procedures, like bone marrow aspirations or port placements in my chest, the songs were recorded in my mind. Instead of scary thoughts, I would quietly sing the music in my mind and the words soothed the fear away.

Books – My sister gave me the first book I received during treatment. Early on, just days after I was admitted into the hospital, she brought me *Why Some Positive Thinkers Get Powerful Results* by Norman Vincent Peale, as a birthday present. I still treasure this book. It helped set my mind to empowerment through strengthening the understanding of managing my own thoughts. It is full of something I knew nothing about at the time: faith-based affirmations. I can't say enough about how impactful this book was in my process.

There were also two other books that became critical tools in keeping my mind straight and my strength solid: *Healed of Cancer* by Dodie Osteen and *God's Promises for Your Every Need* by Jack Contryman, then published in Puerto Rico by Radio Redentor. The latter was a pocket-size booklet. I have seen similar books even in drugstores, although they are printed by different organizations. Every time I was admitted to the hospital, these books came with me.

The benefit of these books is that once I read them, they served as references. When fear, insecurity or exhaustion would try to take over, I could use any of these tools to re-center myself.

Also, the presence of my healing partners was therapeutic. Their love, their jokes and hugs were great at showing me that life was worth fighting for, but for the times my friends and family were not around, they had equipped me with tools like these books and music to help me stay positive and emotionally strong.

There are tools like these for other faiths and philosophies. These helped me even when I was not a traditional believer. If you know your loved one well, you will know what to give her. If not, ask her and others that might be closer to her what might help or simply take a risk and give her what you feel strongly would work. Don't pressure her. Inspire her with your actions.

"Believe, when you are most unhappy, that there is something for you to do in the world. So long as you can sweeten another's pain, life is not in vain."

— Helen Keller

Handling Your Own Emotions

Who are you? Are you a close friend or relative? Are you a spouse or partner? The closer you are to the fire, the more you will feel the heat. The fear, the uncertainty, the pain and the frustration at not being able to wave the illness away will affect you more and more. You need to find a way to come back to yourself, to find some relief. For many of us, the natural instinct is to power through the situation. This feeling may have noble roots, but it can leave you feeling overwhelmed, irritable, angry. You may start snapping at people. In time your emotional condition may deteriorate. This is the opposite of what you want. You are no good to anyone if you break down. As the saying goes, charity begins at home.

Your loved one is not the only one living with the effects of the illness. Your own life is not in danger, but your emotional well-being is under pressure. If you want to help, you also have to help yourself. Here's some advice that can make a difference:

• Make sure you get enough sleep. I cannot emphasize this too much. Sleep is more than resting. It is an active repair process for your body and your brain. Chronic lack of sleep is correlated to dementia later in life[1].

---

[1] https://www.nih.gov/news-events/nih-research-

• Eat well. Don't default to fast food to spend more time with your sick friend. Your body needs the best nourishment it can get, just like hers.

• Pray. Feed your soul. Strength comes from within. This is the time to look for reinforcement not just around you, but from God.

• Exercise. Again, do not allow time constraints to deter you. You don't need to engage in strenuous exercise or exercise for long periods. Studies show[2] that physical exercise is not only good for your body but also for your mind. Exercise can be as effective as anti-depression medication in mild depression cases.

• Go outside. Spend some time in nature. The Japanese term shinrin-yoku, or forest bathing, refers to the practice of walking quietly under the canopy of a living forest. Its adherents say it has many benefits, including:

• Improved immune system function

• Healthier blood pressure

• Lower stress

• Better mood

• Increased ability to focus

matters/sleep-deprivation-increases-alzheimers-protein

[2] https://www.apa.org/monitor/2011/12/exercise

• Higher energy level

• Better sleep

To learn more about shinrin-yoku, visit here: http://www.shinrin-yoku.org or here: https://qz.com/804022/health-benefits-japanese-forest-bathing/

If you don't have a forest nearby, go to the beach. Visit a park. Take your shoes off. Feel the earth beneath your feet in your back yard. Nature has a way of soothing us. Let it.

"So that I may come to you with joy, by God's will, and in your company be refreshed."

— Romans 15:32

Who's Got Your Back?

Elsewhere in this book I have encouraged you to take care of the caregiver. If you're a caregiver, who takes care of you? As we said in the previous chapter, you are no good to anyone if you break down. You need to take care of yourself. In the heat of battle, it's easy to lose track of things and end up shortchanging yourself. This is why it's important to have an accountability partner. This is a friend or partner who will keep an eye on you and remind you when it's time to stop and replenish yourself.

If you don't have a person to fill this position, such as a spouse or romantic partner, you may want to reach out to a friend. It may even be good to approach someone who has little or no connection to your loved one who is sick and is thus not directly involved in supporting her. That way, this person will be able to track your state of mind in a more objective way. This caregiver accountability partner will be able to give you some tough love and stand up to you when you are losing sight of your own needs. This is the person who can grab your arm and take you out for some much-needed *shinrin-yoku*.

Your loved one doesn't need to face her life-threatening challenge alone, and neither should you. Make sure you have someone who will look out for you as you look out for your friend. We all need each other.

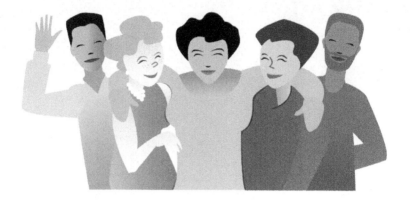

"Be joyful in hope, patient in affliction, faithful in prayer."

— Romans 12:12

Emotions to Expect

You may already be familiar with Dr. Elisabeth Kübler-Ross's framework for the five stages of grief. I know you don't want to think about grieving for your friend. She is alive and fighting to get well. What you may not realize that your friend is grieving.

The moment I received the cancer diagnosis I suffered a loss. I lost the life I had been living up to that moment. I knew that from that moment on, even if I got well, everything would be different. I was right. Don't get me wrong: I am thankful for every day. But the life I had been living ended the day of my diagnosis, and I had to mourn that loss so that I could build a new life. It is the same for everyone. There is no other way.

For you, it is important to understand what your friend is experiencing. Only then will you be able to support her effectively. Only then can you reduce the chances for misunderstandings and confrontations.

I am not a psychologist. Nothing in this section or in this book is meant to take the place of psychological counseling. Counseling is something, by the way, I recommend for you and for your ailing friend. It is beyond the scope of this book to offer an in-depth analysis of Dr. Kübler-Ross's framework. To learn more, read *On Grief and Grieving: Finding the Meaning of Grief Through the Five Stages of Loss,* by Elisabeth Kübler-Ross and David Kessler. Also visit https://grief.com/the-five-stages-of-grief/ .

Dr. Kübler-Ross's five stages of grief are, in order:

• Denial

• Anger

• Bargaining

• Depression

• Acceptance

Let's take a brief look at each.

Denial

Do not worry if your friend tells herself that she's not sick, that her diagnosis is some kind of mix-up or that her illness will go away by itself. Allow her to share her point of view. Ask questions. If she has not sought a second opinion, encourage her to do so. This is temporary. The denial will fade as soon as her mind has had a chance to adjust to the diagnosis. At that point, get ready for the next stage.

Anger

"Why me?" This is the question—or a version of it—people ask themselves after a bad diagnosis. "This is so unfair!" Our notions of fairness and the idea that the world should be fair to us in some way are the source of much suffering in life. If we part the veil of illusion, we can see that bad things happen to good people all the time. No one is trying to punish us. Our illness, to go back to Susan Sontag, is not a metaphor. That said, anger is not entirely a bad thing. It is a necessary emotion that can serve to energize us so we can take action.

Your friend's anger may be all over the place at first. She may lash out at those close to her, including you. Keep this in perspective. She is struggling to come to grips with an overwhelming situation and you may suffer some collateral damage. Be patient. Be kind. This will pass.

Is it fair that you should have to face your friend's anger, when all you're trying to do is help? No. It's not fair. I am sorry, we don't do it consciously or on purpose.

I don't remember ever exhibiting a rage storm, but I remember being in the back of the car as my brother and mother were taking me to the hospital for another appointment. It was one of those days that I was feeling extremely weak. A man that looked much older than me and that we knew was a heavy drug user approached the car to ask for money while we had stopped at a red light. I can recall the incident as if it had just happened a few minutes ago. I thought, *How come he has been out in the streets for years, eating whatever he finds and using drugs, but I am the one fighting for my life?* I just could not understand the logic on that scenario. I hardly drank alcohol, had never used drugs, I had not even tried a cigarette in my life. I was too week to be outraged, but I certainly was disappointed. However, I was blessed that when I expressed my conundrum, my brother did not say anything and my mother just said, "Yo sé, mi amor. Hay cosas que no se entienden." *I know, my love. There are things that don't make sense.*

"I don't want him to get sick," I replied. "I just don't understand how is it possible for him to live a long life like that, but I have to be going through chemotherapy."

They did not try to give me a philosophical or religious explanation, they just let me be. A few minutes down the road we started talking about something else. The image of that paradox dissipated.

Please know that although we might not always talk about it, there is a lot that we process while fighting for our lives. As individuals, we will express those thoughts differently, but we are certainly struggling and are not always capable of expressing our feelings in a healthy way. This is not an excuse, just the truth. Give us space, remember the gift of silence or express empathy, like my mother did.

Bargaining

Every December, thousands make the pilgrimage to the Basilica of Guadalupe in Mexico. They come to visit the image of the Virgin of Guadalupe, said to have appeared to peasant Juan Diego in 1531. They go by car, by bicycle, on foot and even on their knees, some of them carrying statues of the Virgin on their backs. Many of them make the pilgrimage to pay a debt: they made a bargain with the Virgin. They believe the Virgin answered their prayers and now they are paying her back.

The bargain may have been something like this: "If I get well, I promise I will make the pilgrimage to the Basilica on my knees." This kind of bargaining may happen in many ways. It is a reaction to the sense of helplessness caused by the loss. It embodies a desire to regain a sense of power: "If I can make a deal, I can help myself."

Your role is not to pass judgement on this bargaining. If your friend starts going to church after years of not going, or decides to give up sweets, your role is the same. You are there to help and support her with loving kindness. If things go your way, there will be plenty of time to analyze these decisions later.

Depression

This stage can be very difficult for all concerned. At this point your friend may decide there is no point in fighting the disease. Life is unfair. The universe makes no sense. Chemotherapy is torture and the outcome is uncertain. Why bother? We're all going to die, anyway.

The most important thing at this stage is to ensure that your friend agrees to treatment. Many people get over this stage quickly, but others take longer, and there may not be much time to get started.

When the doctor diagnosed me, I was in a bad place emotionally. My boyfriend and I had broken up, I had no children, my job was not fulfilling and although I loved my siblings, they were busy living their own lives. I was lonely, with no particular interest in facing the monumental challenge ahead of me.

The doctors told my family that before considering other treatments, I would have to survive the first dose of chemotherapy. It was not going to be an easy road. I felt all my dreams suddenly meant nothing. I was ready to let go of my life to avoid suffering through the horrors of chemotherapy. Then my best friend sat down with me and gave me a reason to live.

"Do it for me," she said, looking deep into my eyes. "I need you."

That's what brought me back. She brought me back. *Thank you, Mari.*

Every story is different, but I learned one thing: the love of one person can pull another back from the brink of death. If you are lucky, at some point in her journey, you can be that person to your friend.

Acceptance

Acceptance doesn't happen all at once. It happens in stages, over time. It is the winding down of grieving and the start of a new stage. For me, it was the start of the fight, a declaration of war. Against the odds, I declared war on my illness, marshaled my resources, and called on my team. My cancer was already at stage four. I was in big trouble. Today, I thank God I can share this story.

Acceptance can also be of a different kind: accepting that we are looking at the end of the road. This, too, requires courage and grace from your friend and from her support group.

For you, your friend's acceptance of the situation may be the call to join her in her struggle against her illness or to join her as she gallantly prepares for her last goodbyes. Go to her with your heart full of loving kindness. Things are bound to get messy along the way. You're bound to get hurt, but when the journey's over you will know that you would not have changed it for the world.

"Love is not patronizing and charity isn't about pity, it is about love."

- Mother Teresa

Effects of Chemo and Radiation

Chemotherapy and radiation can ravage your friend's body. They can make drastic changes in her physical appearance. This in turn can affect her state of mind. As we have seen before, we should not be too quick to dismiss the feelings of someone who is undergoing this transformation. It is important to reaffirm your love and acceptance for your friend, no matter what changes she experiences in her physical appearance, without minimizing her concerns. This may not always be an easy balance to maintain.

Being too dismissive may lead your friend to say, "That's easy for you to say. You're fine." This may reinforce her feeling that no one understands how she feels, leading her to step back from social contact. That would not be good for her emotional or physical health. Going too far in the other direction may emphasize the negative changes from therapy. That could further depress her mood.

Hey, I never said this was going to be easy!

You may try acknowledging the changes and asking what she wants to do about them, thereby also highlighting she is not totally helpless. For example, you may say, "Yes, I'm sorry you are losing your hair, too. How would you like to handle that until you get your hair back?"

You can also acknowledge the change and reaffirm your feelings for your friend. "Yes, you have lost weight, but I love you no matter what."

There may be no simple solutions, but don't get lost in the details. Keep your eye on the human being you have in front of you. Everything else is incidental. If her depression persists, counseling might help.

Hair Loss

Hair loss is one of the most well-known side effects of cancer treatment, because it is one of the most obvious. As dramatic and hard to handle as it can be, however, it is good to remember that it is usually a temporary effect of treatment. Whatever measures your friend decides to take to manage her hair loss, they are likely to be temporary. The hair will probably grow back later.

Having said that, many people find hair loss depressing. They look at themselves in the mirror and they look so different, that at some level they think, "That's not me." This is disconcerting. In time I came to feel quite comfortable with my bald head, but everyone is different.

Some people opt for using a wig that will allow them to look as close to their pre-baldness self as possible. Others will choose other head coverings, such as hats, turbans or bandanas. Many factors may influence these choices:

• A quality wig that looks natural can be expensive.

• Wigs can be uncomfortable for some people, especially in hot climates.

• Bandanas can be beautiful, but they don't exactly hide the fact that the wearer is bald.

• The same goes for hats. They hide the bald head, but not completely.

The point is that your friend gets to choose whatever works best for her. Your role is to support her choice. This may present fun opportunities if you go hat shopping or wig shopping together. If she chooses to go with bandanas, or hats, this is one more category of present you can offer her. This way, baldness can become an adventure to share, rather than a hardship to endure.

Bodily Functions

The worst time for me during treatment was when my intestines were temporarily paralyzed. The doctors used a tube that went up my nose all the way to my stomach to extract everything from my stomach. I was extremely self-conscious about how odd I was looking. I requested that a dear friend not be allowed in the room because I did not want him to see me looking that way. He made it clear to my family that it was very important for him to be there for me. They asked me to let him come in. I understood that his support was more important than my vanity and I was able to receive the gift of his support.

We have insisted throughout that you should let the patient lead, but there are times when gentle guidance is necessary. No one forced me or made me feel guilty. They just helped me identify priorities.

Weight Changes

Your friend's illness is likely to produce weight loss. Some treatments, such as corticosteroids, may produce weight gain. Depending on your friend's specific illness and treatment, it can go either way. Our culture has an obsession with weight. We promote absurd ideals in the form of altered photographs and video in our media. Considering all this, weight changes can be difficult to manage emotionally.

Here again, your role is to offer acceptance and support. These changes are not the result of your friend's choices. They are the result of her illness and its treatment and there is little she can do about them. Making unsolicited comments about your friend's weight changes is not helpful. If your friend mentions them, be positive and supportive without trivializing her concerns. Like hair loss, these changes are temporary.

Insomnia

Insomnia is much more than a mere annoyance, because sleep is much more than downtime. Sleep in an important active maintenance process for our bodies, including our brains.

Researchers have discovered that the brain flushes out harmful proteins during sleep. These include proteins linked to Alzheimer's Disease. Lack of sleep interferes with this process. This is probably why we find it harder to think clearly when we haven't had enough sleep. Without enough sleep we can also feel overwhelmed and irritable. Insomnia has been found to increase the risk of dementia[3].

Sleep is also linked to weight control. Sleep regulates two hormones that have to do with our appetite. The hormone ghrelin stimulates appetite; leptin decreases it.

3
https://www.ncbi.nlm.nih.gov/pmc/articles/PMC5804010/
https://medicalxpress.com/news/2018-07-disturbances-linked-dementia.html
Wiley. "Optimal sleep linked to lower risks for dementia and early death." ScienceDaily. ScienceDaily, 6 June 2018. www.sciencedaily.com/releases/2018/06/180606082309.htm

When we don't get enough sleep, ghrelin levels go up while leptin levels go down. This leaves us feeling hungry. Lack of sleep also increases levels of another substance called endocannabinoid. This makes us crave carbohydrate-rich foods, like chips and cookies. These foods have low nutritional value and a high caloric content. Translation: they make you fat.

Extended sleep deficits can also affect the levels of insulin and cortisol in our bloodstream. This can result in type 2 diabetes.

You may not be able to lull your friend to sleep, but you may be able to help her establish and maintain habits that can lead to better sleep. Here are some suggestions for all of us:

• Go to sleep at the same time every night.

• Turn the lights out. It may sound obvious, but artificial light can interfere with deep sleep.

• Avoid electronic screens for an hour or two before sleep. If you must use electronics, use an app that will turn the screen to warmer tones instead of the usual cool ones. Cold light inhibits the secretion of melatonin, which helps us fall asleep.

• Exercise regularly, to the degree that you can. Even taking a walk in the evening is good.

• Avoid junk food.

• Learn to meditate. People who meditate tend to sleep better.

• Limit activities in your bedroom. Your bedroom should be for sleeping and making love. And speaking of making love ...

• Have sex. Sex is good for sleep. Orgasm releases a chemical that makes us feel relaxed and sleepy. Your friend might be unable to engage in sexual activity, at least at first. If she is healthy enough to have sex, the prospect of better sleep is another good reason to indulge, if she needs another reason.

Your friend's doctor may also prescribe sleep aids if appropriate.

Tiredness

Both the illness and the treatment take a toll, and your friend will feel tired all the time for a while. There may be times when she'll be strong enough to go out. There will be other times when rolling over in bed will seem exhausting. These are the times when she will not be up to receiving guests or even talking to anyone. She may sleep for long periods or just relax listening to music, reading or watching TV.

Understand that this is part of the process. Don't let your own anxiety get the best of you. Sometimes we want to see our sick friend up and about because that makes us feel better. Remember, this is not about you. Check yourself. If she is awake, watch a movie together. Play cards. Read to her. Listen to a guided meditation together. Or give her some space.

There may be times when the best thing you can do for your friend is to let her be.

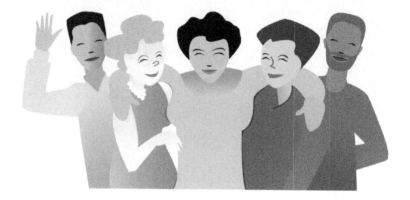

The love of the family, the love of one person can heal.

- Maya Angelou

Other Physical Changes

If your friend requires surgery, the surgery will leave
scars. Endoscopic surgery has made it possible to leave very
small scars in many cases, but endoscopic surgery is not
always an option. Other illnesses, like breast cancer or skin
cancers, can cause more dramatic changes. Some breast
cancer survivors find it difficult to let even a romantic
partner see the scar. Some people find it difficult to look at
their partner's scar.

This is a delicate subject. It is best addressed with loving
kindness and compassion. We all identify with our bodies.
Some say the body is but the temple of the soul, but no one
says, "I live in a brown-eyed body" or "I live in a tall body."
We say "I have brown eyes." We say "I'm six feet tall." We are
our bodies. It is traumatic for anyone to see that she now has
a big scar or that she has lost part of her body. As a spouse
or close friend, your role is familiar by now. Offer support
and optimism without trivializing her feelings. These feelings
may include fear or rejection and shame.

As always, respect her timing. There is no rush. She may
want some time to look at the changes in her body by herself
and get used to it to some extent before allowing anyone else
to see it. Don't crowd her or pressure her. If you find that you
feel uncomfortable with the physical changes in your spouse

or friend, own your feelings. Don't lay them at her feet. Seek professional help. Couples may find counseling useful as they transition into this new stage of their lives. Many other people have gone through this kind of trauma before you. They have overcome the challenge and so can you. There is no shame in getting help.

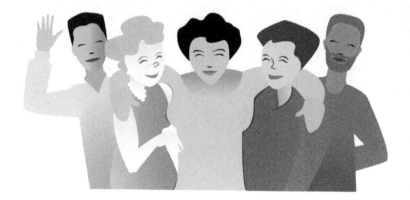

*"As we were
saying yesterday ..."*

- Friar Luis de León

A Parting Word

Friar Luis de León[4] was a Spanish Renaissance poet, mystic and teacher. He was unjustly jailed by the Spanish Inquisition and held for five years. Upon his release he returned to the University of Salamanca, where he was a professor. He started his first class in five years with the now famous words, "As we were saying yesterday ..."

The words are a testament to his character. Friar Luis de León could have come out embittered and resentful. After all, he had spent five years at the mercy of the Spanish Inquisition. Who knows what cruelties he endured. Instead, he chose to put the whole experience behind him and look towards the future. His is an example to consider.

Like the Inquisition, illness is painful. It is all the more painful because it is unfair. It strikes without warning. It robs people of precious time. It hurts the victim's friends and family. It offers no guarantees. As we face this foe, we have a choice to make. Will we allow our bitterness to rule our lives, or will we rise above it?

Whether you are the patient or the friend, whether you win or lose, do not let your pain blind you to the joy and wonder of life. Do what you can to serve today. Fill your

---

[4] Born 1527, Belmonte, Cuenca Province, Spain. Died Aug. 23, 1591, Madrigal de las Altas.

heart with loving kindness. Then give your loved ones the gift of allowing them to help you when your turn comes.

The world is full of beauty.

Be well.

"I don't think of all the misery, but of the beauty that still remains."

— Anne Frank, The Diary of a Young Girl

"Reading is an exercise in empathy; an exercise in walking in someone else's shoes for a while."

-Malorie Blackman

Suggested Reading

In this section you will find other books written for friends and relatives of people facing serious illnesses. These illnesses include different kinds of cancer. Each book is different: each one has its own voice and its own approach.

You will also find books that connect in one way or another to some of the ideas and suggestions presented in this book. For Example, Pema Chödrön's *Living Beautifully With Uncertainty and Change* is a beautiful tool for dealing with the uncertainty that a diagnosis can bring. Kankyo Tannier's *The Gift of Silence* is related to the section in this book by the same name. *Emily Dickinson's Letters* and *The Habit of Being: Letters of Flannery O'Connor* are here because writing letters is one of the suggestions in these pages. These books are fine collections of letters by two notable writers from the United States. Any of these books would be a valuable addition to your library. Good luck on your reading journey.

Chapman, Gary. *The Five Love Languages: The Secret to Love That Lasts.* Chicago, IL: Northfield Publishing. 2014.

Chödrön, Pema. *Living Beautifully With Uncertainty and Change.* Boulder, CO: Shambhala Editions. 2013.

Cornwall, Debora J. *Things I Wish I'd Known: Cancer Caregivers Speak Out.* Sarasota, FL: Bardolf & Company, 2012.

Cottin Pogrebin, Letty. *How to Be a Friend to a Friend Who's Sick.* New York, NY: Public Affairs, 2013.

Countryman, Jack. *God's Promises for Your Every Need.* New York, NY: Thomas Nelson, Harper Collins Publishing. 2006.

Dickinson, Emily. *Emily Dickinson's Letters.* Mabel Loomis Todd, Ed. New York, NY: Dover Publications. Reprint edition (June 26, 2012).

Drescher, Fran. *Cancer, Shmancer,* New York, NY: Grand Central Publishing, 2002.

Frankl, Victor E. *Man's Search for Meaning.* New York, NY: Beacon Press. 2006.

Kalick, Rosanne. *Cancer Etiquette: What to Say, What to Do When Someone You Know or Love Has Cancer.* Scarsdale, NY: Lion Books, 2004.

Kneece, Judy C., RN, OCN. *Helping Your Mate Face Breast Cancer: Tips for Becoming an Effective Support Partner for the One You Love During the Breast Cancer Experience.* West Columbia, SC: Educare, 2003.

Kübler-Ross, Elisabeth; Kessler, David. *On Grief and Grieving: Finding the Meaning of Grief Through the Five*

Stages of Loss. New York, NY: Scribner, Reprint Edition. 2014.

O'Connor, Flannery. *The Habit of Being: Letters of Flannery O'Connor.* Sally Fitzgerald, Ed. New York, NY: Farrar, Straus and Giroux. 1988.

Osteen, Dodie. *Healed of Cancer.* Houston, TX: John Osteen Publications. 1986.

Peale, Normant Vincent. *Why Some Positive Thinkers Get Powerful Results.* New York, NY: Open Road Media. 2015.

Sontag, Susan. *Illness as Metaphor.* New York, NY: Farrar, Straus and Giroux. 1978.

Tannier, Kankyo. *The Gift of Silence: Finding Peace in a World Full of Noise.* London: Yellow Kite. 2018.

Weiss, Mark S. *When Your Wife Has Breast Cancer: A Story of Love, Courage & Survival.* New York, NY: Ibooks, 2006.

"The roots of all goodness lie in the soil of appreciation for goodness."

-The Dalai Lama

Acknowledgements

I could write another book with pages filled with gratitude. I will be brief, although the feeling is boundless.

I am thankful to God, the source of all that is good. His mercy and love shone through all those who were by my side and brought me back to life. That love flooded my mother's heart. It strengthened her body to be by my side every single day of every treatment, every appointment and every day of bad news, until the good news came along. Thank you *Mamita Santa*, for all the sacrifices you made.

That same love guided my brother, Roberto González Rivera. He became a beacon of light illuminating the path to the best treatment available and the culmination of this book of love applied. To my brother José Arnaldo González and his wife Miriam, thank you for showing me with your actions what faith looks and feels like. You strengthened my soul, which in return strengthened my body. The gift you gave me is eternal and priceless. Thank you, my sister, Maritza González. You made time when you did not have any and reminded me that I was still me. Thank you for your beautiful and practical gifts. Thanks to my aunt Perla Rivera and all my Ponce cousins for the radio marathon and much more. I must also extend my gratitude to my cousin, Barbara Rapp. You turned your home into the "command center" to coordinate all supporting activities and then turned it around to host Holiday celebrations. The food, the music, the love, they all brought great joy to the family during our must difficult times. Thank you!

My friends ... I could not ask for better friends. Mari, Lourdes, Nellie, Ivonne, Carlos. You were there e-v-e-r-y day, every way you could. Thank you Glorimar Yace, Rafi Muñoz and Janet Hassinger, my angels in Texas. Thank you all. I felt your presence then, and your kindness is forever imprinted on my heart.

Thanks also to my other friends and family members who let the love of God lead your actions. You were my companions, drivers, sources of laughter and loving distraction and fundraising executives. Many thanks, Rosita Gandía for moving heaven and earth in Arecibo. Thanks to Minerva González and her whole wonderful family. Thank you, thank you, thank you.

Special thanks to Celina González, Amanda Tarkington, Barbara Reynolds, Mitzi Voracheck, Conne Ward-Cameron, Julie MacFarlane, Mari Cidre, Lourdes Arbelo and Carlos Fournier. You took time out of your busy lives to read the manuscript and provide thoughtful feedback. This book is much better because of you.

And finally, my gratitude to an Island full of kind, generous hearts, Puerto Rico. Some of you knew me and some of you did not, but you supported me all the same. Thank you for sending me letters with encouragement and funds for my treatment. Your hand-written envelopes carried more than dollars. You included blessings, prayers, Bible verses, and good wishes ... Your words were a balm to my heart. To all, *muchas gracias*. Thank you!

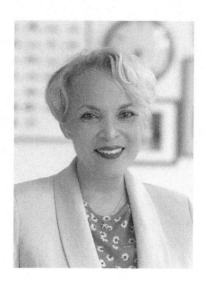

About the Author

Belsie González, MPH, is a two-time leukemia survivor. She is a public health professional passionate about empowering others through information, especially those who are not often seen or heard. After the experience of fighting for her life, she is sharing the lessons she learned so others can make decisions based in information and compassion, not fear.

Belsie has a master's in public health and has worked in that field for more than 20 years. She currently lives in Georgia surrounded by nature. She is available for public speaking engagements in English and Spanish. You can reach her at BelsieGonzalezAuthor@gmail.com.

If you enjoyed this book, please consider taking a moment now and leaving a review on Goodreads (https://goodreads.com) or with your online retailer so others can discover it.

Made in the USA
Monee, IL
30 November 2021

83489268R00105